HOMEOPATHY AT A GLANCE

An Encyclopedia of Safe and Effective Remedies

Margit Wendelberger-James
(MA, Cert.Ed., RSHom)
(Registered Homeopath)

B. Jain Publishers (P) Ltd.

First Edition Sept. 1997
Reprint edition 2001, 2002

Price: Rs. 35.00

All rights reserved with the Publishers
Without limiting the rights under copyright reserved above, no part of this publication may be reproduced, stored in or introduced into a retrieval system, or transmitted, in any form or by any means (electronic, mechanical, photocopying, recording or otherwise), without the prior written permission of both the copyright owner and Publishers of the book.

Published in India by:
B. Jain Publishers (P) Ltd.
1921, Street No. 10, Chuna Mandi,
Paharganj, New Delhi-110055, INDIA.
EMAIL: kjain@giasdl01.vsnl.net.in

Printed in India at:
J.J. Offset Printers
7, Wazirpur Printing Press Area,
Ring Road, Wazirpur, Delhi-35

NOTE FROM THE PUBLISHERS
Any information given in this book is not intended to be taken as a replacement for medical advice. Any person with a condition requiring medical attention should consult a qualified practitioner or therapist.

Book Code : **BM-5244**
ISBN: 81-7021-803-X

CONTENTS

I   Introduction 5

1.1   The history and tradition of homeopathy 7
1.2   Vital principles of homeopathy 9
1.3   How homeopathic remedies are made up/
      "potencies" 10
1.4   Does homeopathy work?
      The scientific argument in favour of homeopathy 12
1.5   What makes homeopathy so special? 14

II   Homeopathy for self-treatment 15

2.1   How to take homeopathic remedies 17
2.2   The step-by-step
      guide to finding the correct remedy 20
2.3   Trouble-shooting:
      Common questions answered 24
2.4   Where to obtain quality remedies/
      How to find professional help 27

III Caution - limitations of self-help 29

      1)   Aconitum napellus 31
      2)   Allium cepa 33
      3)   Apis 35
      4)   Arnica montana 37
      5)   Arsenincum album 39
      6)   Belladonna 41

7)	Berberis	43
8)	Bryonia	45
9)	Calendula	47
10)	Cantharis	49
11)	Carbo veg.	51
12)	Chamomilla	53
13)	Cocculus	55
14)	Gelsemium	57
15)	Hypericum	59
16)	Ipecac	61
17)	Lachesis	63
18)	Ledum	66
19)	Mercurius sol.	68
20)	Nat. sulph.	70
21)	Nux. vom.	72
22)	Paeonia	75
23)	Pulsatilla	77
24)	Rhus. tox.	80
25)	Ruta grav.	83
26)	Symphytum	85
27)	Urtica urens	87
28)	Veratrum album	89
V	Index of Conditions and Symptoms	93
VI	Bibliography	96

HOMEOPATHY -

The concise step-by-step guide for successful home treatment

Introduction

Homeopathy has been used for nearly 200 years to cure illness safely and efficiently, with gentle speed and ease. Its appeal lies in its holistic approach - the whole person is treated, the focus is *"the person, not the cure"*. It therefore offers a real alternative to pharmaceutical drugs, which concentrate on pathology only. These are expensive and often carry the risk of unwanted side effects, whereas homeopathic remedies are non-toxic, without accumulative effect, yet at the same time are a *safe and gentle* way to improve your health permanently.

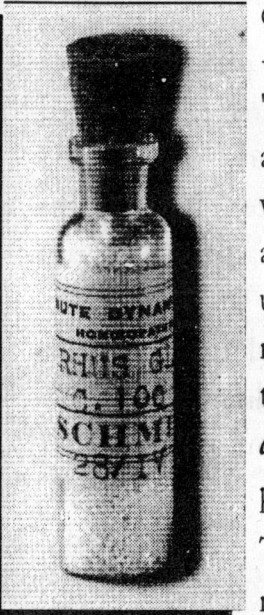

The Royal Family has for a long time recognized the health benefits of homeopathy. In 1835 Queen Adelaide, Queen Consort of William IV, received successful homeopathic

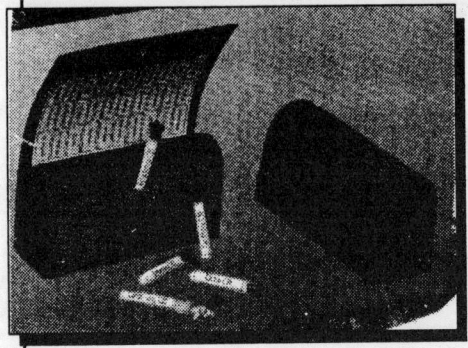

treatment and thereby started an intimate friendship between homeopathy and the Royal House. Maybe this accounts for the good health and the longevity of the House of Windsor!

Today the Queen Mother is Patron of the British Homeopathic Association and Queen Elizabeth is Patron of the Royal Homeopathic Hospital in London.

This book sets out to give you the tools to prescribe at home for yourself, your family and friends. All the remedies described are clearly labelled and categorized. By using the key characteristics of each remedy you can obtain successful results in treating minor diseases, acute illnesses and emergencies.

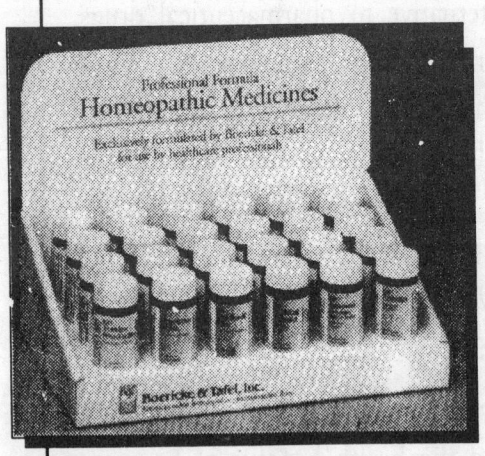

Please read section II carefully before starting out treating yourself and others as it contains valuable advice on safe prescribing.

1.1
The history and tradition of homeopathy

Homeopathy can rely on a long-standing tradition. Homeopathic ideas already circulated at the times of the great Greek physicians, yet lacked the coherence and systematic approach that was later established in the early 19th century. As early as 400 B.C. Hippocrates identified two methods of cure, one by "*contraries*", the other by "*similarities*", the latter being the major principle of homeopathy.

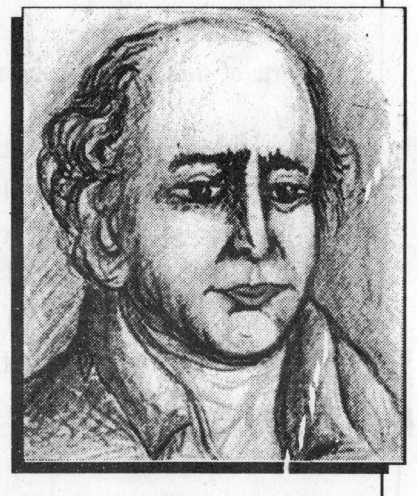

This distinction is based on the notion that a fever for example may either be cured by administering fever reducing drugs such as salicylic acid, the main component of "Aspirin", which is the way of contraries. On the other hand Belladonna or Aconite may be given, which in small portions cause a feverish illness in *healthy people*, yet in true fevers help to cure the patient by "*similarities*", which is the central idea of homeopathy, i.e. "*like cures like*".

The most prominent figure connected with homeopathy, however, is Samuel Hahnemann, the late 18th century German physician, who "discovered" homeopathy by self experiment. In 1790 he took a quantity of cinchona or Peruvian bark. He thereby tried to prove that this plant cured intermittent fever and allayed the ill person's suffering, by causing symptoms similar to the one created by the disease.

> *Like Cures Like*

He determined that, cinchona, from which later quinine was derived for the treatment of malaria, brought on malaria symptoms in the body.

Hahnemann reasoned that a substance which produced certain effects -symptoms- in a healthy person, may cure the same symptoms in a sick person. The most central idea of homeopathy, the "*law of similars*", was born.

Samuel Hahnemann researched and consolidated his findings for almost 20 years before in 1810 he finally published his theory in a coherent form in the Organon der Heilkunst (*Tool of the Art of Healing*), which caused quite a stir among the medically trained practitioners and pharmacists at the time.

> *Organon*
> *Tool of the Art of Healing*

The idea that *like cures like*, in addition to the claim that a minute, "inert" dose of a substance may cure serious disease seemed paradoxical as well as controversial and has continued to attract criticism and derision even today.

1.2
Vital principles of homeopathy

As we have seen, the law of similars is a central notion of homeopathy. Another one is that only one remedy at a time should be administered. This is to facilitate monitoring the effect of the remedy and thereby to make vital decisions about the course of the treatment.

In addition, "classical" homeopathy, which follows the strict guidelines in the tradition of Hahnemann, stipulates that only the least possible amount is required to heal, a rule which makes sense given the excessive drugging with crude substances that patients were subjected to in the 18th century. (It is open for discussion if this policy has really changed fundamentally since the days of Hahnemann...)

> Law of
> Similia
> Simplex
> Minimum

By using the smallest possible dose to cure a disease, the self-healing potential of the body is activated and stimulated. The body thereby learns to efficiently deal with the disturbed body function without the detrimental side effects of pharmaceutical drugs.

This was exactly Hahnemann's aim when he set about to find a system which gently and efficiently assisted the body in dealing with a particular disease. He was vehemently opposed to creating drug induced illnesses in his patients, caused by the severe side effects of the drugs prescribed. Sadly side effects in modern pharmaceutical drugs are also common today.

1.3
How homeopathic remedies are made up/ "potencies"

Usage of the minimal dose requires an intricate process of dilution and succussion (shaking) of the original substance, which can be of animal, plant or mineral origin.

Dilution involves reducing the strength of the original tincture ("mother tincture") or solid mixture by adding purified, distilled water in the case of fluids, lactose (milk sugar) in the case of solids.

As soon as the strength of the tincture of mixture has been adjusted to the requirements, the potion is shaken ("succussed") and the solids are ground in a mortar. This process is called potentisation and today in Britain we have a scale of potencies ranging from 6c to 1M, 10M or even 50M.

For our purposes we shall only be looking at the "c" potencies ("c" for centesimal), as they are best suited for home treatment. "C" potencies indicate that to 1 part of medicated mixture there has been 99 parts of carrier (alcohol, water or lactose) added, one part of this mixture is again diluted with 99 parts of the carrier substance etc. We therefore find increasing dilutions in homeopathy which represent the different "steps" in potencies.

This process is repeated in the centesimal potencies as many as 3, 6, 12, 30, 100 or 200 times. As the final result we have 3c, 6c, 12c, 30c, 100c or 200c. These potencies should suffice for home treatment, as they are perfectly safe in your hands, given that certain guidelines and rules are observed, please refer to chapter 2.1 "How to take homeopathic remedies".

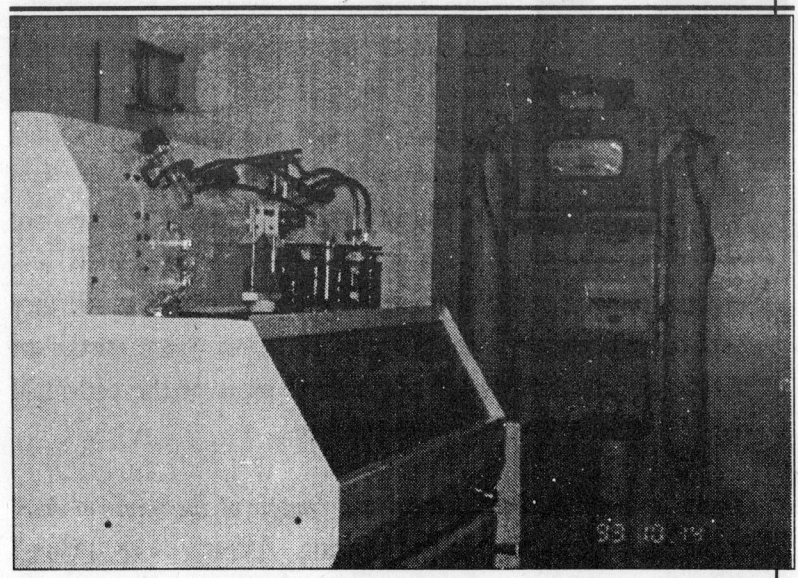

1.4
Does homeopathy work?

The scientific argument in favour of homeopathy

Conservative science claims that homeopathy cannot work, except for a certain placebo effect between prescriber and patient. Yet it works perfectly on babies, small children and animals, where the placebo effect thanks to belief and trust in the prescriber and the remedy is absent. Why?

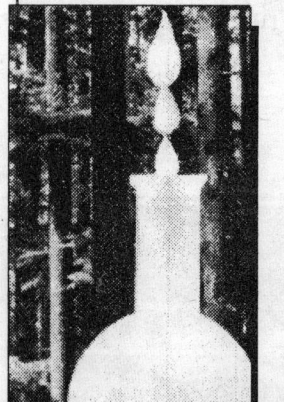

It is true that in potencies from 12c and above there is no evidence of molecular presence of the original (medicated) substance. We are merely left with the molecular make-up of the diluent water, alcohol (ethanol) or lactose. It seems probable that the diluent acts as a magnetic tape, not unlike a video tape, which has recorded and thereby "remembered" the properties of the original substance they have been in contact with. These properties or characteristics act beneficially on the physical and mental plane of the patient, if the remedy has been skilfully matched.

There is scientific evidence for the *"magic of the minimal dose"* or the principle of dilution to extinction. As early as 1930 Cotell conducted tests on cats and frogs, exploring the efficiency of different dilutions on the organism. One of his extraordinary findings was that even a tiny amount of acetylcholine was able to lower the blood pressure of the animal. (1)

More recently, in 1988, Dr Jaques Benveniste, a research director with INSERM, the French national medical research, carried out experiments with very dilute solutions of antiserum added to blood. When certain types of blood cells come into contact with antiserum, they are destroyed. (2)

1) The ratio of the dilution was one miligram to 500,000 gallons of liquid. (Everybody's Guide to Homeopathic Remedies, Cummings and Ullman, 1986, p.15.)

2) The Sunday Telegraph, article by R. Matthews, 3rd July 1994

Dr Benveniste claimed that antiserum-free, "activated" solutions destroyed almost as many of the blood cells as the original antiserum. This seems to support the thesis that water is able to retain a "memory" of the properties of the antiserum, even though there are no molecules of the original substance present in the diluent.

Perhaps not surprisingly, Dr Benveniste was told in 1993 to terminate his experiments which could have been a sensational breakthrough for homeopathy, as they suggested that water has an electromagnetic "memory".

However, even without complete scientific validation it is clear that homeopathy works. It is a safe, gentle and efficient alternative to pharmaceutical drugs and it will work for you for the benefit of yourself and your family.

1.5
What makes homeopathy so special?

First of all homeopathy is prescribed for the individual and not for the individual symptom. The motto "*the patient, not the cure*" shows how homeopathy cares for the particular patient and his unique physical and mental/emotional make-up.

By treating the whole person as an entity it achieves better, more comprehensive and long-lasting cure than conservative, drug based medicine.

Secondly, in homeopathy only very small amounts of a medicated substance are used. These remedies are safe and gentle even for children and babies as they are non-toxic and have no unwanted side-effects. No animal experiments have been carried out for the production of homeopathic remedies.

Finally and most important, homeopathy aims at strengthening the body's natural defence system and thereby increasing one's resources. There is a tendency to self-healing in all of us and only when our defences are down, when we are "off colour", can micro-organisms find an entry and cause disease. These self-healing powers are encouraged and strengthened by homeopathic treatment instead of being obstructed or even paralysed, which is the effect of most pharmaceutical drugs.

Treating yourself homeopathically will not only help you to recover more quickly and efficiently from illness, but will also provide you with more energy and zest in life.

I believe you will enjoy reading this book, as it provides invaluable information about the best used homeopathic remedies, together with advice and guidance on self-prescribing in most first aid situations and for home treatment in general.

2
Homeopathy for self-treatment

Homeopathy aims to treat the whole person, not just the disease. In order to self-treat successfully one must learn to distinguish the guiding symptoms or "key notes" which characterize a remedy and accordingly distinguish it from another.

For successful prescribing at home you should aim to find at least three symptoms which can be associated with any particular remedy in this book. Particular attention should be given to any mental/emotional symptoms, like "wants company","angry" etc.

You will find "pointers" to the remedy at the end of each chapter on one particular homeopathic preparation. Each remedy is easily identified by looking at the single bullet point for each characteristic. Your aim should be to find three matching characteristics for each prescription.

Using the pointer scheme plus your observation skills, objectivity and

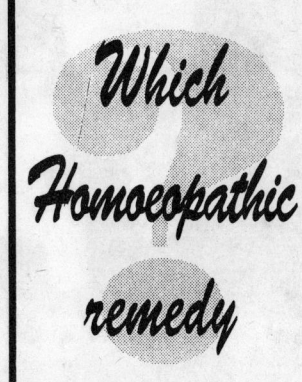

patience will yield excellent results for you when prescribing for a patient.

An example for good homeopathic prescribing is when a child comes home hot and bothered *first symptom*, with a sharp rise in temperature towards the evening *second symptom* together with flushed, hot skin *third symptom* and aggravation from being touched and moved *additional fourth symptom*.

These three "key notes", ie characteristic, main symptoms, plus a confirming fourth symptom, denote a remedy particularly suited for feverish conditions, *Belladonna*.

As far as the potency in the above example is concerned, according to the severity of the symptoms the prescriber would give a matching potency, in this case probably a 30c. As a rule of thumb it can be said that the stronger the symptoms and the faster the development of the disease, the higher the potency should be to match the high energy curve of the illness.

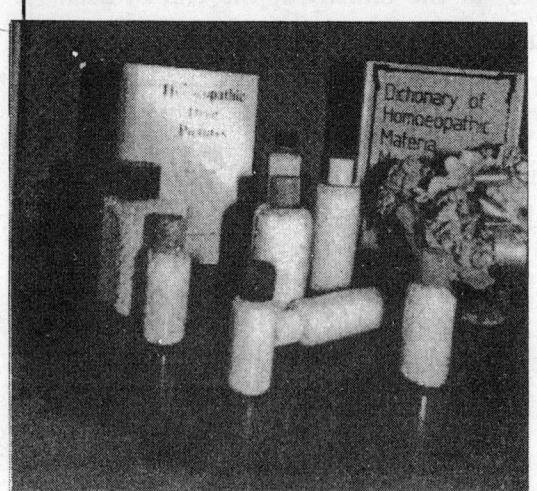

2.1
How to take homeopathic remedies?

In acute situations with a fast developing display of symptoms taking the indicated remedy may be necessary every half an hour until the symptoms decrease and the patient feels better in him/herself. When the remedy works and there is an evident improvement in the patient's condition you can leave larger gaps between each dose according to the reaction of the body.

Should no reaction to the remedy occur within the space of half an hour to an hour the remedy choice has been erroneous and needs to be changed.

Which potency? How often

Children and babies usually show a very good and clear reaction to an indicated remedy. If the child is very small a liquid remedy is preferable or the remedy in the form of a tablet should be crushed or dissolved in water and then be given. The same applies for pets. If the patient is unconscious you can wet his/her lips or tongue with the liquid remedy in small amounts. However, it is also of paramount importance to refer the person to a medically trained professional.

Remedies can also be added to food or drink, but it is preferable to take them on their own, letting them dissolve in the mucous membranes of the mouth. While taking homeopathic remedies strong smelling substances like coffee, camphor, menthol,

How to obtain best results

peppermint and eucalyptus oil (toothpaste!) should be avoided, as they can interfere with the action of the remedy.

This also applies for today's popular aromatherapy oils, of which the strong smelling oils like camphor, peppermint and eucalyptus should be avoided.

Usually the correct remedy will help very quickly and only a single or one second dose will be necessary. If there has been some improvement after the first and second dose but the problem has not yet resolved itself completely, you can continue taking the remedy as long as improvement occurs.

Should no further improvement occur and the health problem is considerably better but not fully resolved, it is best to wait for a day and then reconsider the case and examine the remaining symptoms.

Make a list of the still persisting symptoms and refer to the index section to see if a new remedy has emerged. If that is the case a new remedy will continue the good work for the benefit of the patient.

In any case please abstain from finishing the whole bottle of the remedy without reassessing your symptoms and the improvement in your health after a day, latest a week after commencing a remedy.

People have been known to take a particular remedy for years because it helped them initially. *This is not good for your health as you may eventually display symptoms of the remedy.*

For example "Sulphur" may originally have helped you with a rash which was very itchy, red and made worse by contact with water. After months of taking the remedy you may find your skin becoming coarser and drier, and your hands and feet have started to feel hot and burning, particularly at night.

These are exactly the symptoms that Sulphur has been known to cause in healthy volunteers. As you may have taken this remedy over a considerable length of time your body has started to "take on board" some of the symptoms of the Sulphur "picture".

What originally helped you with your skin rash has now outdone its good work by subtly introducing Sulphur symptology into your body system.

It is important that you only take remedies with caution and respect and that you don't overdose just because "they are natural and can't do any harm". Although they cannot actively poison you, the molecular amount of active ingredient being too minute, they can cause you discomforting new symptoms instead of clearing up troublesome old ones.

If you have tried several remedies to no avail it is worthwhile reconsidering your prescribing and the conditions under which the remedies have been taken, or seek the help of a professional homeopath (see chapter 2.4 on how to find a good homeopath).

You may wish to observe the following points in your quest for the ideal remedy.

2.2
The step-by-step guide to finding the correct homeopathic remedy

1. **Observe the patient carefully.**
   This includes examining the skin colour and temperature, body temperature, sweat, body odour, etc. How does he/she interact with his/her environment?

2. **Question the patient on his/her condition.**
   Ask him/her how he/she feels about him/herself. What makes him/her feel better or worse, including environmental influences (temperature, time of the day, other people's company and concern etc.) and food and drink (how much, how often, preferences?).

3. **Write down the key information.**
   It is best to have a short and concise list of symptoms, with at least three characteristic items.

4. **Look in the index under the appropriate heading.**
   For example under the general heading "colds and catarrhs" you

How to monitor your successful prescribing

will find several remedies. Go to the appropriate remedies and read the general information on each remedy. This will give you a broad idea about the type and character of the remedy.

5. **Look up the indicated remedy "characteristics".**
   Compare your list with the summarized list of "characteristics" at the end of each remedy.

6. **Make your remedy choice by comparison.**
   Once you have found among the characteristics some remedies which are close to the condition you are trying to treat, read the portraits of the indicated remedies. Particular attention to the "Therapeutics and Indications" section should be given, as this covers the homeopathic application of the remedy. You will now have arrived at one, possibly two remedies as your final choice. Select the remedy which is most appropriate before deciding on the potency, bearing in mind the second remedy as further possibility should the first one fail.

> Three symptoms of your list and the listed symptoms of a certain remedy should ideally be identical.
>
> Please note that you should only select one remedy as your final choice, not giving two remedies at the same time, even if they are close. This safeguards better monitoring and evaluation of your treatment.

7. **Decide on the potency.**
   Acute conditions, especially in the first two days, need

potencies in the range of 30c to 200c, depending on the severity and strength of symptoms. Children respond well to remedies and usually need lower potencies, it is a good idea to start with a 30c.

Example: Head cold, 1 day. Patient feels very heavy and lethargic, can hardly keep his eyes open, small of the back aches, he/she is running a slight temperature. Prescription: Gelsemium, 30c, every other hour until better.

Please remember that chronic conditions, with a duration of half a year or longer, need potencies below 30c. The same applies if you are very sensitive to any form of treatment, are allergic to certain substances, pregnant, elderly or convalescent. Children should be started on 30c as they usually react very quickly and strongly to homeopathic treatment.

8. **Check your remedy kit if you have the remedy and potency available.**

9. **Administer the remedy in the appropriate way.**

    Leaving a 20 minute gap between any food or drink and the remedy, also avoid coffee and other strong smelling substances such as peppermint tea/oil.

10. **Wait and observe.**

    Wait at least 1/2 hour in very urgent, acute cases (with a lot of pain or discomfort) to one or two days in long-standing, chronic health problems.

11. **Before prescribing the next dose check with the patient if there has been an improvement or other change.**

    Go back to your list and compare again with the "pointers" of the prescribed remedy. Is the remedy still indicated? If yes you can give a second dose. If not, compare the list with other possible remedies.

    Please go to chapter 2.2 "Trouble-shooting" if you have any doubts about the course of your treatment.

    This process may seem lengthy, especially when treating an emergency, but observation, careful assessment and patience are essential to good homeopathic prescribing.

    After you have become used to the process it will become second nature and become faster, the reward being accurate, successful homeopathic treatment.

    Furthermore, after you have prescribed the same remedy various times and you have developed a "feel" for the remedy, you can probably shorten the selection process by just checking the keynotes with the "pointers" of your pre-chosen remedy. Eventually you may even prescribe well-known remedies from experience, as you will probably know the remedy by heart.

2.3
Trouble-shooting – Common questions answered

Remedy taken................No effect

Have you antidoted with coffee or other strong smelling substances? This may reduce or eliminate the beneficial effect of a remedy.

Have you eaten or drunk something immediately before or after a remedy? This may reduce its action.

Have you made your selection with at least 3 good symptoms? Otherwise your prescription may be too speculative.

Have you waited at least 1/2 hour after the remedy before assessing the effect of the remedy? Otherwise you may be too confused to get good, clear symptoms to prescribe on.

How attached are you to the patient?

If you are emotionally involved it might be better to ask another person to assess the effect of the remedy, as being objective is a key factor to good prescribing.

Have you tried a different potency, usually higher than the original one, for example 200c instead of 30c?

This will release more energy than the 30c and might be more appropriate to the condition you are trying to treat, especially in acute illness.

FINALLY:

Have you tried a different remedy yet?

Remedy taken……..some success but not yet fully recovered

Have you taken at least 2 doses of the remedy? Maybe you should take another dose (max. 3)

Perhaps you ought to be more patient. Waiting for a few days can help to mobilize your vital force and increase your own capacity for self-healing.

Remedy taken……..only partial improvement after a sufficient period of waiting

Have you waited long enough? Minimum half an hour in acute conditions, at least a day in health problems of long-standing nature. Chronic problems with more than half year's duration can take several weeks to respond, so after an initial dose of 3 homeopathic tablets you may want to wait a week to a fortnight to reassess your improvement in health.

The rule is the longer you have suffered with a particular ailment, the longer it will take to cure it with homeopathic remedies.

On the other hand, if you are trying to treat a chronic condition your knowledge of homeopathy may not be sufficient. It is best to get some advice from an experienced homeopath.

Have you reassessed your symptom picture, i.e. have you made a list of what has changed, what has remained?

It is best to have a tangible list as it will help your remedy choice.

Have you compared your list with the list which prompted you to choose the first remedy?

Does it still fit the remedy? If not you may need a new remedy.

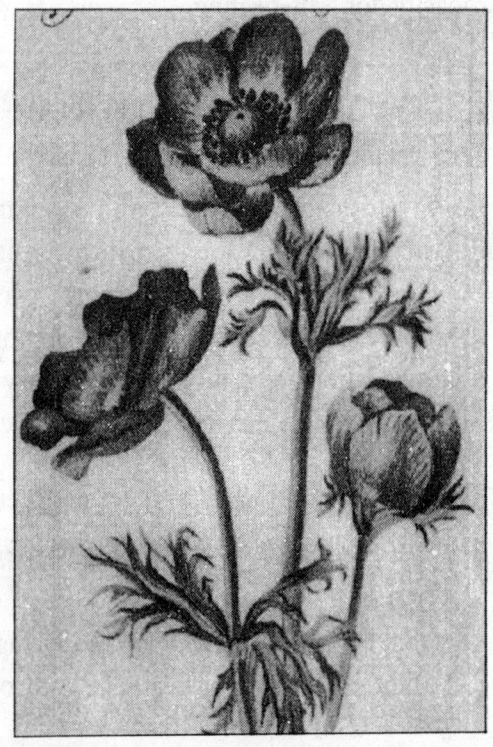

2.4

Where to obtain quality remedies/ how to find professional help

Remedies can be procured at most chemists and health food shops, although they mostly stock common remedies and low potencies (6c), together with some homeopathic ointments. For different potencies and more unusual remedies please see your local dealers, selection of the right supplier is very important.

At last a word of caution - chronic disease should best be left to the experienced, professional homeopath, as it is probably too complicated and entrenched to be treated by the self-prescriber. Equally if you get "stuck" with your self-treatment and the symptoms are not improving or are actually getting worse it is recommended that you seek professional help.

Medical emergencies should be referred to a medical doctor, in addition to homeopathic self-help.

Please see the next chapter for a clear definition of emergency situations.

3
Caution – Limitations of Self-help

General symptoms

Unconsciousness; severe bleeding; continued vomiting and diarrhoea; severe concussions; fractures; high fever (102F/39C or higher) over more than 3 days.

It is vital to know the limits of one's own self-prescribing and to recognize possibly life threatening emergency situations.

Calling a doctor or referring to casualty is recommended when the following symptoms occur:

Specific symptoms

- severe breathing difficulties with dizziness, cyanosis (*blue discolouration*); [*blocked airway?*]

- pain in the chest with nausea, vomiting, sweating and fear [*heart attack*]; colicky pain in the navel region, patient feels nauseous, might have foul breath, followed by severe pain in the lower right abdomen if pressed gently and then released [*appendicitis*];

In babies under 6 months the following symptoms should give cause for concern:
- Not feeding for 12 hours,
- Floppy,
- Sunken eyes,
- Lethargy or irritability,
- Unresponsive,
- Loss of fluids for 6 hours or more

- stiff neck, photophobia (aversion to light), fever and a rose-red rash on the buttocks and thighs [*meningitis*];

With older children, please refer to casualty in addition to a homeopathic remedy in the following situations:

>   Bleeding which cannot be stopped
>
>   Internal bleeding, the child looks pale, is possibly confused, external bruising, he/she may complain of pain
>
>   A deep wound with debris or an object embedded
>
>   A deep puncture wound from a knife or nail
>
>   An animal bite
>
>   A significant electric shock
>
>   A major burn or scald
>
>   Loss of consciousness
>
>   Any suggestion of poisoning
>
>   Choking should be treated instantly by removing the object from the larynx

However, with some common sense and growing confidence these emergencies will be recognized and handled with ease. Most minor complaints can be treated successfully with homeopathy by the home prescriber, if you follow my recommendations you should recognize your limits in prescribing for emergency situations and chronic illness.

> **You should Recognise your limits in presenting emergency situations**

Aconite (Plant)
(Aconitum Napellus)

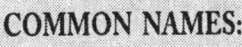

COMMON NAMES:
Monkshood, Friar's cap, Wolf' Bane

Description: A poisonous perennial, which grows to 3 ft. in height with dark blue flowers.

Habitat: Grows wild and in the garden. One of the rare true blue garden flowers, Aconite prefers moisture retentive soil and grows best in light shade.

Medicinal Action and its Uses: The highly poisonous alkaloid of the plant, found in its root, causes circulatory disturbances such as numbness, tingling, shivering and burning. The victim of such a poisoning dies of circulatory paralysis and cardiac arrest.

Therapeutics and Indications: Aconite is of great benefit in fevers and colds/flu which come on rapidly, often after exposure to cold, dry winds, and which are swiftly followed by a sharp rise in temperature. The patient feels chilly and resents noise and touch. In the evening the symptoms (fever, chilliness and red hot skin) are especially pronounced. Peculiar is that the patient has a pronounced fear of death, he/she is sure they will die from this illness, they even predict the day. In children there is simply fear and although the child may not be able to voice the particular nature of this fear, he/she may cling to their carers for support and reassurance.

Potency and Dosage: As usual in acute cases and particularly in this remedy, Acon. 100c to 200c should be given initially. A dramatic improvement in symptoms such as reduction of the fever and of the sensation of burning and heat, should be expected rapidly. Once improvement has set in, a lower dosage and potency is recommended, indeed a repetition may not be necessary at all.

It is important to remember that giving the remedy once as in Acon. 200c should drastically reduce the symptoms and lead to rapid improvement and recovery.

Characteristics to remember:

- Patient has fever, with an acute rise in temperature, particularly in the evening
- The skin looks red and is hot to touch
- He/she feels chilly
- Patient sweats profusely
- He/she dislikes noise, touch and warm rooms
- The symptoms appear very rapidly in otherwise healthy people
- There is a peculiar *fear of death* although the illness itself may not be life-threatening

Allium Cepa (Plant)
(Allium Cepa)

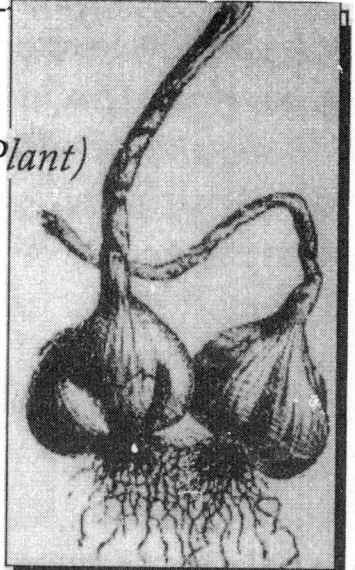

Description: The red onion is a popular vegetable. Most people are familiar with the red bulb, which is revealed on cutting white flesh with purple, concentric rings.

Habitat: Onions need fertile, well-drained soil and plenty of sunshine. They are cultivated commercially as well as in the pottager of the hobby gardener.

> **COMMON NAMES:**
> *Red Onion*

Medicinal Action and its Uses: Allium cepa is an antiseptic and diuretic. It has traditionally been used for treating viral infections of the upper respiratory tract. Half a cut onion placed in the room where the patient rests, can act as a helping agent in troublesome coughs. Onion syrup (macerated onion mixed with sugar, left to infuse and then drained) has been used for the same purpose.

Therapeutics and Indications: Allium cepa is a very effective homoeopathic remedy for catarrh of the upper respiratory tract, especially for nasal discharge. This discharge is usually acrid and invokes a burning sensation to the upper lip and wings of the nose. In contrast, discharge from the eyes is bland.

Catarrhal headache can also occur with this type of head cold, which is worse in warm rooms. A typical All. c. cough is set off by breathing in cold air, there is also tickling in the back of the throat.

Characteristics to remember:
- Bland discharges from the eyes
- Burning discharges from the nose
- Conditions worse in the warm surroundings
- Cough brought on by inhalation of cold air
- Useful remedy in hay fever

e patient feels generally better outside in the open air. A cool room is also appreciated. Evening can be particularly aggravating for the All. c. patient.

As with an ordinary cold the same symptoms can appear in hay fever. This remedy has been proven to be very effective in annual hay fever which follows the symptoms as described above.

Potency and Dosage: Depending on the severity of the symptoms, a lower dose (6c to 30c) mornings and evenings for a few days will usually be very effective.

Apis (Animal)
(Apis Mellifica)

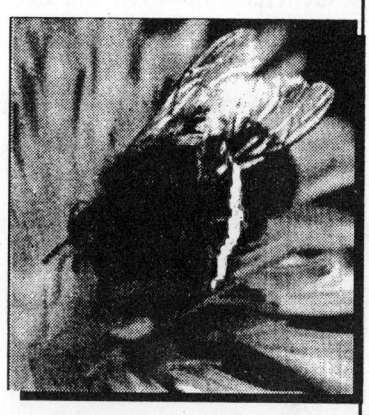

Description: The honey bee (Apis mellifera) is an industrious, sociable animal with the ability to produce excellent nourishment (honey, pollen, royal jelly). At the same time it is capable of producing a poison which produces pain and swelling of the human skin. The honey bee forms large colonies with one queen bee, several hundred droves and 50,000 to 80,000 workers. The bee society is complex, with a caste system and strictly defined tasks for the different member groups.

Habitat: Although there are several type of bees: mining bees, carpenter bees, bumble bees, orchid bees, stingless bees and honey bees it is predominantly the latter which is kept and managed for their honey production in gardens and on farms.

COMMON NAMES:
The Honey Bee

Medicinal Action and its Uses: The effects of a bee sting on humans are well-known: burning, stinging, with reddening and swelling of the affected parts. Some people are hypersensitive to the bee poison which can result in anaphylactic shock or collapse with difficult breathing and sudden drop in blood pressure.

Generally, however, the bee sting leaves little effect other than discomfort and swelling.

The poison from the bee sting has been used medicinally to treat rheumatism and other forms of joint pain.

Therapeutics and Indications: Apis is derived from the bee poison, released in the bee sting. Not surprisingly Apis is an excellent remedy for insect bites and stings, especially when caused by horse flies, wasps or bees. Children and sensitive adults (although not people suffering from bee sting allergies) will benefit greatly from this remedy, when an insect bite causes great discomfort, with puffy swelling and burning pain.

Potency and Dosage: One dose of Apic 6c will usually soothe the sting and remarkably reduce the uncomfortable effects of the insect poison. Repeat 6c if necessary.

Care should be taken if the individual, especially when a child with multiple insect bites shows signs of general distress, such as pallor, nausea, gross swelling and/or the appearance of a rash. You can use Apis 30c or 200c in such cases, but also seek medical advice immediately.

Characteristics to remember:

- Stinging and burning pain with swelling of the affected body part after insect bites
- Puffiness of the affected area
- Patient dislikes touch and heat in any form
- Cool compresses and cold bathing of the affected part affords relief

(A little vinegar in the water will help to reduce the swelling externally)

Arnica (Plant)
(Arnica Montana)

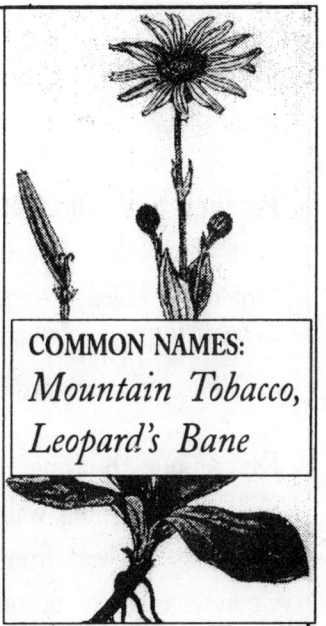

COMMON NAMES:
Mountain Tobacco, Leopard's Bane

Description: A perennial herb, growing to 1 ft high, the flower being bright yellow.

Habitat: Grows on mixtures of loam, peat and sand. The herb is native to the lower mountain slopes of northern and central Europe.

Medicinal Action and its Uses: Arnica has long been recognized for its superb action in shock, concussion and bruises due to falls and other accidents. Continental Europeans always made use of its beneficial effect on soft tissue injuries, the German speaking countries for example calling the herb "Fallkraut" (Tumble weed). The first reference to the medicinal action of Arnica was made by Hildegard of Bingen in the Middle Ages.

Therapeutics and Indications: Bumps and bruises of all kinds, notably to the head (*concussion*). Excellent first aid remedy for shock (*accidents*). Arnica can also be given prior to or after operations, including dental treatment and post partum (*childbirth*). It is used in heart attacks, when the patient is conscious.

People who need Arnica dislike touch and motion and feel better lying down.

Potency and Dosage: In accidents and severe bruising Arnica should be taken internally, 200c, every half hour, in milder cases 30c or 100c, only one dose or two.

For minor bruising and over exertion (gardening, walking, muscle strain derived from unusual/vigorous exercise) 6c or 12c, one dose or two, will afford relief.

Concussion and bruising can also be successfully treated with Arnica ointment, applied liberally on the affected area and repeated for several days. Mother tincture (the plant extract) can be used for the same purpose, but has to be diluted, 5 drops to 1/2 pint of water, for the use as a compress.

Care should be taken not to use Arnica on broken skin, as it can cause a skin reaction in sensitive people.

Characteristics to remember:
- At least 3 of these pointers to the remedy should be found in the patient
- Use in shock and trauma after accidents or injuries (physical or psychological)
- Patient feels bruised
- There are externally visible bruises
- Sensation of being weary and exhausted
- Conditions worse from movement and exertion, also from skin contact
- Conditions worse from exposure to the sun and/or damp cold
- Patient has sprained and dislocated feeling in the joints
- Bed feels too hard, difficulty getting into a comfortable position

Arsenicum Album (Element)
(Arsenicum album)

Description: Organic arsenic compounds were used as the first effective pharmaceutical drug against syphilis, developed by Paul Ehrlich at the beginning of the 19th century.

Medicinal Action and its Uses: Ars. is an excellent remedy for digestive upsets, food poisonings and gastroenteritis.

COMMON NAMES: As, element 33. A grey metalloid in the nitrogen family, used in some lead alloys. White arsenic (arsenicum album) is arsenic III oxide (As_2O_3), has been used in rodent control and in poisonings.

Therapeutics and Indications: Gastric disturbances together with the following general symptoms call for the remedy: restlessness, lack of vital heat, feeling worse at night. The patient feels weak and exhausted. The digestive symptoms are very specific: There is increased thirst for frequent, small quantities of drink, the sight or smell of food causes nausea; stomach pains are burning and there is diarrhoea which is offensive in smell and often dark in colour.

Mentally the patient fears the worst, that he or she has a very serious disease or is even about to die. Generally there is much anxiety about one's state of health.

Potency and Dosage: In severe cases, especially while travelling abroad, Ars. 200c once whilst fasting and rest should bring enormous relief. The symptoms should improve and cease altogether within 1-2 hours of taking the remedy. Thereafter repetition may not be necessary, but if some symptoms persist, repeat with a lower potency, 30c or 6c. In less severe cases, start the treatment with Ars. 6c or 30c.

It is generally better to give one dose of Ars. 200c and to wait for a few hours before deciding whether a repeat remedy is necessary.

Characteristics to remember:
- In mild or severe cases of food poisoning or consumption of "borderline" food
- Anxious patient, he/she fears the worst about his/her health
- He/she "hugs" the fire or other sources of heat
- He/she vomits and/or suffers from offensive diarrhoea
- Excessive thirst prevails, mostly for cold drinks, little and often
- Restless, he/she cannot keep still and rest although exhausted

Care should be taken to avoid dehydration, the patient should drink plenty of fluids, as they may have lost a lot of body fluids.

Extra tip: Ginger tea helps to overcome gastric upsets. See p.60 (Ipecac) on how to prepare the tea.

Belladonna *(Plant)*
(Atropa Belladonna)

> **COMMON NAMES:**
> *Devil's Cherries, Black Cherry, Devil's Herb, Deadly Nightshade*

Description: Perennial plant, 3 to 5 ft high, with dull green leaves. The flowers are bell-shaped of dusky purple colour. In September the small, black berries develop which are juicy and intensely sweet. The fresh plant, when crushed, gives off an unpleasant odour.

Habitat: It prefers fertile, chalky soil and dappled shade, ideally on the forest floor.

Medicinal Action and its Uses: Herb and root are used for medicinal purposes. They contain an alkaloid which render the plant very poisonous. The effects are inhibition of glandular secretion, i.e. dry mouth and reduction of sweat. Bell. relaxes muscle cramps, it therefore is given by the medically qualified in colics and angina pectoris. Bell. is furthermore used in ophthalmology (eye treatment) and as an antidote to some poisonings.

Therapeutics and Indications: Bell. is a fine remedy for the treatment of flu and fever, which develop quickly and intensely. The patient is hot to touch, positively radiates heat and has red, shiny skin. There is internal burning and pulsating heat, the sufferer resents light, motion and drafts of cold air. Children may have horrible dreams and hallucinations. Sufferers improve in warm conditions. This is a remedy which should also be considered in sunstroke.

Characteristics to remember:
- Use in acute fevers and flu
- Victims of sunstroke may benefit from the remedy
- Patient radiates heat
- Skin is hot, red and shiny
- Patient resents light, touch or movement
- Tongue is strawberry colour
- Thirst for lemon juice, lemonade or similar drinks

Potency and Dosage: Bell. conditions develop quickly and therefore will hardly require more than one dose of Bell 200c. Repeat the remedy if only a partial recovery has been achieved with Bell. 30c. If the patient is weak, dissolving the tablet in a glass of water and asking them to drink small sips at frequent intervals will prove very beneficial.

Berberis (Plant)
(Berberis Vulgaris)

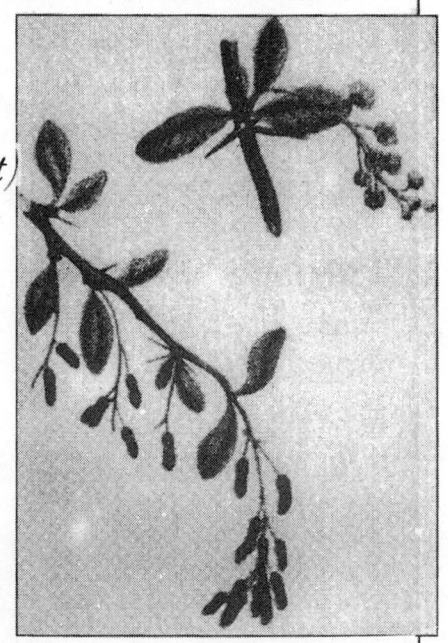

COMMON NAMES:
Barberry,
Pipperidge Bush

Description: A shrub of 8 to 10 ft in height with ash coloured bark. The flowers are pale yellow in colour and have a disagreeable smell. The berries, produced in autumn, are bright red and taste acidic, as do the leaves.

Habitat: Originally a wild shrub found in hedges, the barberry is now grown in gardens and farms. It requires sun or semi-shade and any free draining soil. It is attractive to gardeners for its fruit and colourful autumn foliage. Pollinating insects are also attracted to the multitude of small flowers.

Medicinal Action and its Uses: Berberis is used to treat constipation and also for liver disease, but only by qualified herbalists.

Therapeutics and Indications: In homeopathy, Berberis is used for cystitis and bladder problems, and is also used to treat kidney- and gallstones. Cystitis is the most likely condition to be treated at home. The symptoms are: burning pains with a "never finished" feeling after urinating. The pain extends to the thighs and the groin. The colour of the urine can vary from pale to deep yellow, even with a reddish tint. There maybe also some bran-like sediment and gelatinous, "slimy" matter in the urine.

Characteristics to remember:
- In bladder inflammation with burning, smarting pain
- "Never finished" feeling after urinating
- Urine has a different colour and appearance from normal (paler/darker/reddish tinge)
- Urinary pain extends to the thighs and the groin

Potency and Dosage: In acute conditions Berb. 30c will suffice when taken regularly at 2 hourly intervals until the pain and the other urinary symptoms have subsided.

Bryonia (Plant)
(Bryonia Alba)

Description: A vine-like plant with a climbing habit, the tendrils of which attach themselves to their support. This plant is related to the cucumber and shares its hairy, deeply cut, five-lobed leaves and stems. Bryonia produces small white-green flowers in spring and pale scarlet berries in autumn which are unpleasant in smell. The whole plant tastes acrid and bitter.

Habitat: Bryonia grows abundantly in hedgerows and woods in Southern England and Southern Europe. It likes dappled shade and moisture retentive soil.

Medicinal Action and its Uses: In herbalism, the fleshy root is used as a strong purgative and as a cathartic to clear out the digestive tracts.

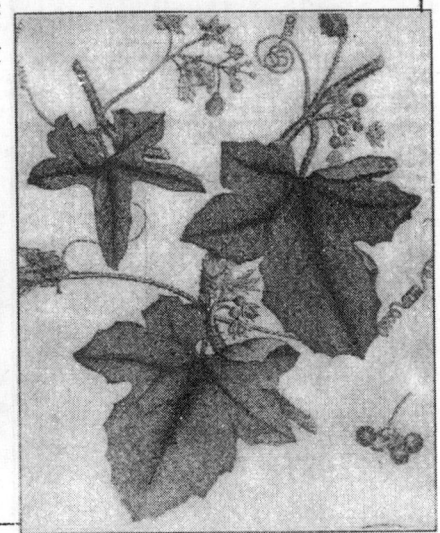

COMMON NAMES:
Wild Hops,
Wild Vine,
English Mandrake

Therapeutics and Indications: Bryonia is an excellent remedy for bronchitis and pneumonia, where the cough is irritable and dry, with dry mucous membranes. Coughing is painful to the degree that the sufferer crosses his/her arms in front of the chest to ease the strong pain. When coughing, the patient wants to sit up. Movement is very painful and any form of movement at all, i.e. physical movement, movement of the surroundings (the bed), even mental movement (thinking) causes distress. Rest and hard pressure on the affected areas affords relief.

Characteristics to remember:

- Use in "dry" infections of the bronchi and lungs
- There is little or no sputum brought up by coughing
- Membranes of the mouth/throat are dry
- Any form of movement disturbs and aggravates
- Patient resents warmth, touch and being spoken to, but welcomes hard pressure to the affected area, as in lying on the affected side and quiet rest

Potency and Dosage: In acute bronchitis Bryonia 200c brings instant relief. This dose possibly has to be repeated the next day or, if substantial improvement has set in, Bry. 30c can be used as a follow-up. In pneumonia and/or dry pleurisy (inflammation of the membrane containing the lungs) 30c, given at regular intervals every 2-3 hours will be very beneficial.

Calendula *(Plant)*
(Calendula Officinalis)

Description: A plant which is 10-20" in height, the marigold is a familiar sight in the garden. It is an annual which self seeds very easily. The light green leaves distinguish themselves from the bright yellow-orange flowers which are reminiscent of the midday sun in their clarity, shape and cheerful colouring. The flowers are pleasantly bitter to taste and aromatic in smell.

Habitat: The plant is easily grown in almost any soil but it prefers a sunny, sheltered position.

Medicinal Action and its Uses: Marigold is used in creams and ointment for topical skin application. The herb was considered to be beneficial

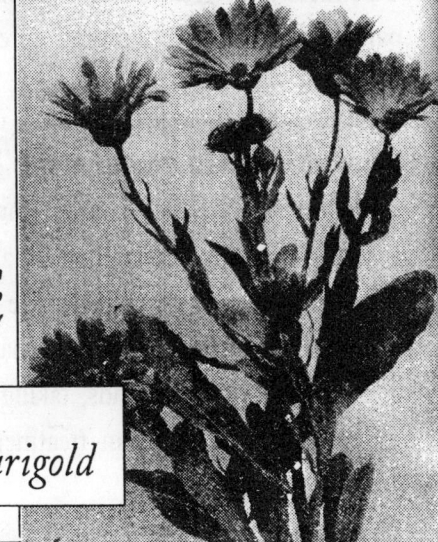

Marigold, the source for Calendula officinalis. The whole plant is used to make the remedy

COMMON NAMES:
Marigold, Pot Marigold

in liver conditions. For everyday purposes Marigold flowers are rubbed into the skin to bring relief from insect bites.

Therapeutics and Indications: Calendula is of outstanding value as a skin remedy. Ragged, torn or inflamed wounds are very easily treated with a topical application of Calendula ointment or a medicated compress/plaster. Similarly after operations, in dental surgery or childbirth a topical application of Calendula is of great benefit. It swiftly helps to heal the injured part of the skin and prevents infection.

Characteristics to remember:
- Use in skin lesions where the skin has been broken, i.e. in cuts, grazes, surgery
- Apply externally, for smaller wounds as ointment, for bigger wounds as a compress
- In large wounds support external treatment by giving Calen. 6c twice daily
- One of the most useful remedies for home treatment

Potency and Dosage: Calendula ointment and mother tincture is available for skin treatment, the latter has to be diluted 1 part of tincture to 50 parts of water (or a few drops per pint) before application as a compress. For smaller wounds ointment is most appropriate. For bigger wounds the diluted remedy is best applied as a moist gauze compress and changed before the compress has dried out. In large wounds, taking Calendula 6c twice daily in conjunction with the skin treatment will speed up the healing process.

Cantharis *(Animal)*
(Cantharis Vesicator)

Description: A slender, metallic-green beetle which exudes acrid yellow fluid from its joints.

Medicinal Action and its Uses: Wing cases of cantharis vesicator were collected for their "cantharidin", a blistering agent. Spanish fly has been used as an aphrodisiac to increase sexual passion. This has led to many cases of fatal poisoning, due to the high toxicity of the substance.

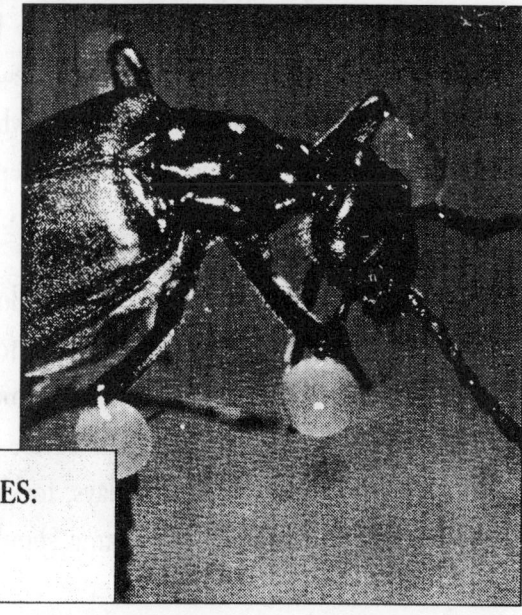

COMMON NAMES:
Spanish Fly

Therapeutics and Indications: Cantharis, the homoeopathic preparation of the whole insect, is used for cystitis and bladder problems. These are characterised by a great amount of cutting and burning pains from the kidney to the bladder and down to the sphincter. Passing urine is accompanied by violent cutting and burning pain, as if "molten lead" is being passed. The desire to pass water may or may not be increased, but the actual act causes a feeling of scalding when the bladder is emptied. The urine is pale yellow or deep red, with bloody discharges.

Characteristics to remember:

- Use in cystitis and urinary infections
- Burning and cutting pain before and after urination
- Feeling as if molten lead is passed
- Pelvis and bladder region are extremely sensitive to touch, which the patient resents

Potency and Dosage: In severe cases one dose of Canth. 200c will bring immediate relief. This can be followed by 30c the next day and thereafter, depending on how much discomfort is still felt. In minor cases with less severe symptoms and less pain, Canth. 30c on subsequent days, for 3-4 days, will bring about a speedy recovery. This regime should also be followed if Canth. 200c is not available.

Carbo Veg. *(Plant origin)*
(Carbo Vegetabilis)

COMMON NAMES:
Charcoal

Description: Charcoal is a form of carbon made by heating vegetable substances (mostly wood) in the absence of air, which drives off the volatile constituents. It is very porous and absorbs 90% of gas before saturated, hence its use as an absorbent and filter.

Medicinal Action and its Uses: Charcoal tablets are given for diarrhoea and in gastro-enteritis, as their high absorbency guarantees that some of the bacteria invading the gut is absorbed and rendered harmless.

Therapeutics and Indications: The main sphere of action for Carbo veg. is the digestive system. Although there is a craving for greasy and rich food, it tends to upset the patient. He/

she feels generally worse after eating, especially fatty food. Digestive symptoms include: heartburn, indigestion, belching, flatulence and griping stomach pain. The patient feels cold and weak, with extremely cold extremities including a cold nose and knees.

Characteristics to remember:

- Use in digestive problems, especially with a lot of flatulence

- Patient feels weak, very cold and sluggish

- Bad reaction from fat foods, especially butter

- Patient cannot bear any tight clothes around the waistline

- Relief is obtained from being fanned, fresh air and cool wind

Potency and Dosage: Carb.v. 6c or 30c will help in the above type of gastric upsets, taken daily for 2-3 days. After this the remedy can be continued for another 2-3 days if there is good improvement yet not a complete cure.

Chamomilla (Plant)
(Chamomilla)

Description: Low growing plant with hairy and freely branching stems. The leaves are fine, divided into feathery-like segments. The small, white and golden flowers display a bright yellow centre like a conical cushion and the flowers give off an aromatic, apple-like scent.

Habitat: Chamomile grows in fields, on rubble heaps and along fences and hedges. It prefers plenty of sunshine and light soil.

Medicinal Action and its Uses: Chamomile has been used since ancient times for stomach upsets and generally to soothe and relax. It is used as a hot

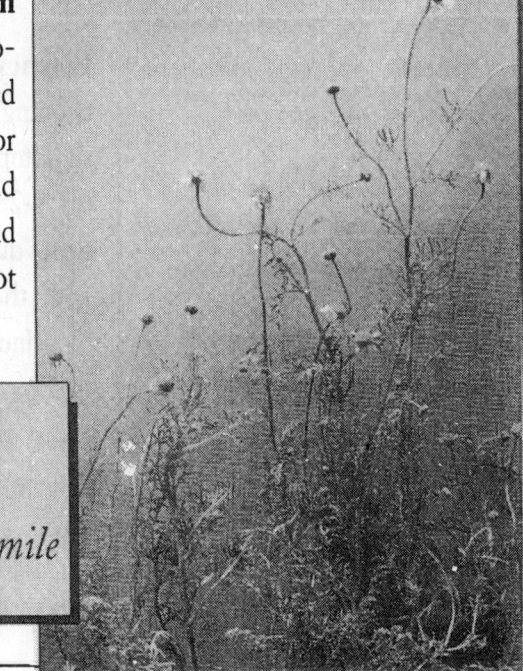

COMMON NAMES:
Chamomile,
Common Chamomile

steam sauna for the face and for gargling. The latter is beneficial in abscesses and boils as chamomile greatly reduces the swelling and inflammation. In aromatherapy a dilution of chamomile oil is used for sprains.

Therapeutics and Indications: Chamomilla as a homoeopathic preparation is excellent for children's teething problems and tantrums. The child displays extremely bad temper and tantrums with the physical symptoms. He/she cannot be pleased or comforted and there is a lot of angry crying. In teething problems one cheek is red hot while the other is cold. Toothache is worse after hot drinks. Earaches can generate much soreness and ringing in the ears. External heat (e.g. hats) can drive the patient to distraction.

Potency and Dosage: Depending on the severity of the symptoms, Cham. 6c to 30c, for 1-2 days twice daily will bring quick relief to the child and the exhausted parent. Continue with 6c for a maximum of a week if symptoms have not completely vanished after the initial two days.

Characteristics to remember:

- Physical symptoms with bad temper: snappy, impatient, whining and restless

- Excellent children's remedy and in menstrual or pregnancy problems with bad temper

- First remedy to consider in children's teething problems

- Aggravation from heat, open air, touch and contradiction

- Patient feels better when carried or driven around

Cocculus *(Plant)*
(Cocculus Indicus)

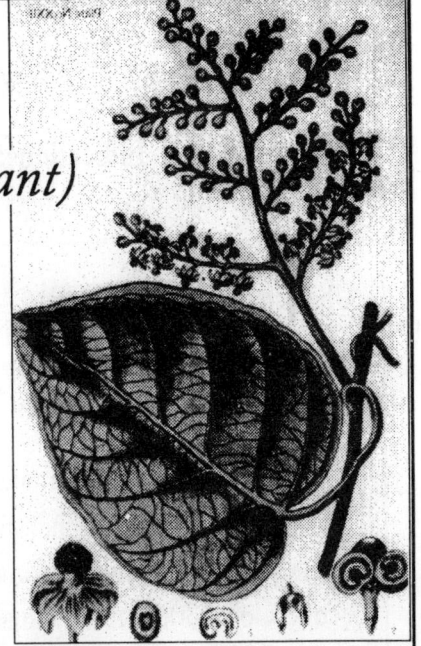

COMMON NAMES:
*Indian Cockle,
Levant Nut.*

Indian cockle, the source for Cocculus indicus. It was proved by Hahnemann and appears in the third volume of his Materia Medica Pura

Description: A poisonous climbing plant with ash-coloured bark and smooth, heart-shaped leaves. The fruit is kidney shaped, brown-black and wrinkled, inside are two white seeds per "nut" which are very oily. The latter contain the poisonous substance picrotoxin which is responsible for the medicinal action of Cocculus Indicus.

Habitat: A plant of the Southern hemisphere, indigenous to India, Sri Lanka and Malabar.

Medicinal Action and its Uses: Apart from its mundane use by fishermen of stupefying fish by throwing the whole fruit in the water, Cocculus Indicus has been used with moderate success in checking night sweats of TB sufferers.

Therapeutics and Indications: Cocc. can be used in home prescribing to treat travel sickness and jet lag. Cocc. has an affinity to the sense of hearing and balance, and as this is disturbed when travelling on a plane, bus, boat, car or train, the remedy is of excellent value in such cases.

Nausea, headache and vertigo is common in travel sickness and Cocc. can give enormous relief if the complaints are worse from movement, cold air, eating and drinking. Jolting and jarring movements can make the patient feel worse. In jet lag, Cocc. is used when the traveller feels exhausted and cannot sleep, the biological clock being disturbed and upset.

> **Characteristics to remember:**
> - Use in travel sickness and jet-lag
> - As preventive treatment take Cocc. 30c two days before the journey commences and one Cocc. 30c on the actual day of travel
> - In acute attacks of travel sickness, take Cocc. 30c every hour until the symptoms subside
> - Bachflower remedy "Clematis" is also reknowned to prevent or ease the symptoms of travel sickness
> - Put 2 drops of "Clematis" in 1/2 glass of water and take small sips or in emergencies put two drops directly on the tongue

Gelsemium (Plant)
(Gelsemium nitidum)

COMMON NAMES:
Yellow Jasmine, Carolina Jasmine, False Jasmine, Wild Woodbine

Description: Gels. is a climbing plant from the Southern States of North America. It possesses great climbing power, often ascending several feet onto trees and spreading an equal distance with its fleshy roots underground. The flowers are funnel-shaped, of yellow color and emit a delicious scent.

Habitat: This is a plant of southern climes, preferring the moist and warm atmosphere of the Southern States of the US. As a vigorous climber it often reaches 10 ft or more, scaling trees in the search of sunlight. To appreciate the beauty of the flowers and their scent, Gels. can be grown under glass in cooler climates.

Medicinal Action and its Uses: Gels. contains two deadly alkaloids, Gelseminine and Gelsemine. These are extracted from the roots of the plant. The drug is a potent spinal depressant, which targets the respiratory centre of the medulla oblongata, the lower part of the brain stem. Death occurs by depressed and ultimately arrested breathing.

Gels. has been used as a treatment for various types of fevers, among them malaria and swamp fever. Whooping cough and asthma have also been successfully treated with Gels.

Therapeutics and Indications: In homeopathy, Gels. is used for flu/colds and feverish conditions. They are of a particular slow nature and are characterised by a feeling of heaviness (heavy limbs, heavy eyelids) and languor. The patient wants to rest in bed and sleep, every effort is resented because of an all pervading weight on the body and spirit. To summarise: "Apathy reigns supreme".

Headaches with feverish conditions are "heavy" and dull, the patient feels too exhausted to lift the head from the pillow. The face is flushed and hot, perhaps with a dusky hue. The eyes are swollen and the eyelids are heavy.

Characteristics to remember:

- Particularly in summer colds and flu
- Chilliness runs up and down the spine
- Everything feels heavy and slow
- Colds come on gradually
- The patient feels apathetic and listless

The symptoms are made worse from: the heat of the sun, damp weather, cold, fog and thinking about oneself. The patient is better from open air, gentle continuous movement and bending forward.

Potency and Dosage: High, fast fever spikes are not to be expected with this remedy, as it takes on a slow pace in developing. Gels. 30c, once or twice daily, depending on the severity of the illness, for 3-4 days, will bring the patient quickly on the road of recovery.

Hypericum (Plant)
(Hypericum Perforatum)

Description: A herbaceous perennial, Hypericum flowers faithfully every year. The 20-50cm stem splits into several smaller stems, carrying perforated ("perforatum") pale green leaves. The bright yellow flowers appear from May to August, they exude a resinous smell and are studded with small cells containing blood-red oil.

Habitat: Hypericum likes uncultivated ground as in the vicinity of hedges, wild meadows and woods. Dry ground and sunshine are the preferred situation.

Medicinal Action and its Uses: Following the Doctrine of Signatures - the medieval belief that a plant which resembles a certain organ will cure the same - St John's Wort was used for wounds and for menstrual disorders. The perforated leaves point to its use as wound treatment. The English herbalist Culpepper also recommended St. John's

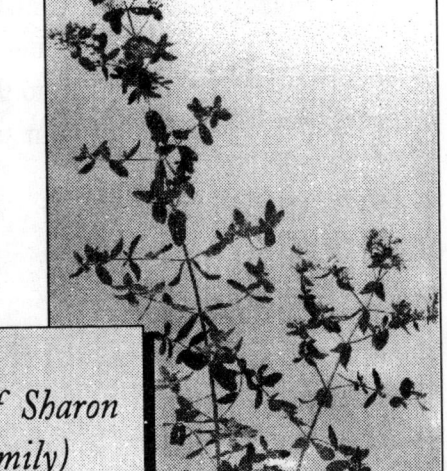

COMMON NAMES:
St. John's Wort, Rose of Sharon (as one genus of the family)

Wort for tuberculosis.

Today there is some interesting research taking place into the properties of Hypericum as a treatment for depression and AIDS.

Therapeutics and Indications: Hyper. is a fine remedy for the treatment of lacerated and punctured wounds. In the latter case it is often used in the conjunction with Calendula tincture as in "Hyper-Cal", a combination of both remedies. Interestingly, Hyper. prevents tetanus infection of wounds treated with the remedy.

Furthermore Hyper. is indispensable for injuries to nerve rich areas, such as crushed fingers and toes, or an injury to the base of the spine. Puncture wounds to the palms of the hands or soles of the feet benefit greatly from treatment with Hyper.

Hyper also finds its use in post-operative treatment, especially in amputations.

Potency and Dosage: Apply as an ointment or a diluted dressing to the wound. This should be a dilution of 5 drops per 1/2 pint of water.

Characteristics to remember:

- Excellent in wound treatment, especially in combination with Calendula

- For nerve injuries: crushed fingers/toes, injured spine or head

- Prevents tetanus

- Patient feels worse for touch and exposure to cold

- Used as an ointment or diluted as a compress

Ipecac (Plant)
(Ipecacuanha)

COMMON NAMES:
Ipecac root

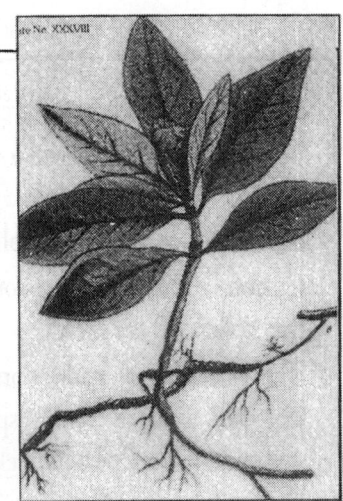

Description: A shrubby perennial plant about 1 foot high whose roots resemble a string of beads. The leaves of the plant are oval and the flowers are small and white.

Habitat: The plant grows in moist, shady woods and is a native of Brazil, Granada and Bolivia. The roots are collected in January and February and then dried in the heat of the sun.

Medicinal Action and its Uses: The root provides the drug Ipecacuanha, used to induce vomiting and to treat dysentery. The nature of the plant is reflected in the native American name, which literally means "roadside sick making plant". The plant extract has been used to induce vomiting and in smaller quantities as an expectorant (to clean the passageways of the lungs) and in even smaller quantities as an appetite stimulating drug.

Therapeutics and Indications: Ipecac's strongest indication is in nausea, especially in pregnancy ("morning sickness") and when young children are sick. The nausea is persistent, accompanied by vomiting which does not relieve. The sufferer is thirstless and has a clean tongue. He/she vomits food, bile, mucous, blood or a combination of all four. Food is rejected and ejected, literally.

Diarrhoea may also be present, with continuous urging to stool.

Children produce grass-green, foamy and copious stool.

Mentally and emotionally the patient is dissatisfied. Everything appears lacklustre, even repugnant, which finds its ultimate expression in the severe physical nausea.

Curiously there can be bone pains with the nausea, especially of the bones of the head.

The suffering is made worse from lying down, moist warm wind and cold weather. Food, especially veal or pork also aggravates the symptoms. The person feels better in the open air.

Generally the subject is chilly and shudders from the slightest cold air or reduction in temperature.

Potency and Dosage: In acute nausea, Ipec. 30c once daily for 2-3 days or until full recovery has been achieved is recommended.

In persistent cases, for example "morning sickness" where homoeopathic treatment has only been started after a number of "sick" days, Ipec. 6c, once a day for a week, will prove to be gentle and even more effective than Ipec. 30c.

Extra tip: Ginger tea also helps to overcome nausea, including morning sickness and general gastric disturbances. To make the tea, slice a fresh ginger root into 5-6 thin slices and simmer for about 15 minutes with a mugful of water. Strain and serve to calm the stomach and quell nausea.

Characteristics to remember:

- A remedy for persistent nausea with vomiting

- Vomiting does not relieve the symptoms

- The sufferer is often thirstless and always chilly

- Cold and moist/warm weather aggravates the patient

- Repugnance for food and life in general

Lachesis *(Animal)*

(Lachesis muta)

Description: Lachesis muta is a rare pit viper and the largest poisonous snake in the New World. Lachesis muta is native to Central and South America, it can grow to a length of 11 1/2 ft and it shows a orange and black pattern on its skin. This snake is a nocturnal animal which spends the hot hours of the day in the cool and moist shade of the forest. It eats small mammals, even small deer, which it fixates with its gaze before killing it. When

COMMON NAMES:
Poison of the jungle snake
Surukuku or Bushmaster

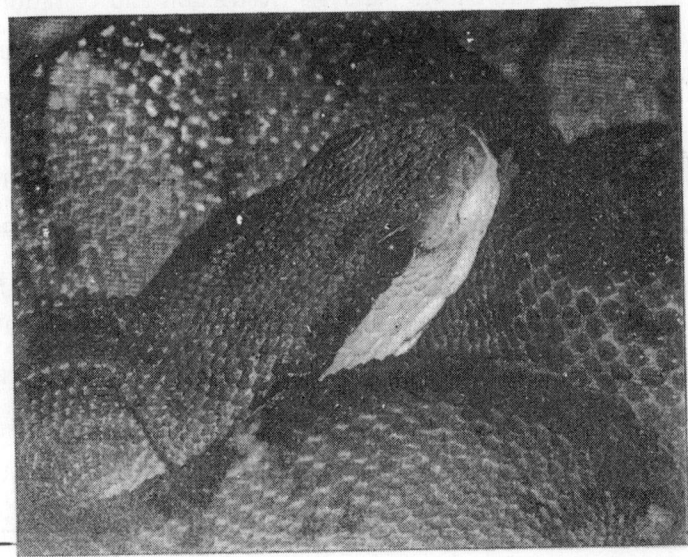

Characteristics to remember:

- For the treatment of sore throats and female problems
- Use in menstrual problems which are relieved with the start of the period
- Aggravated by heat and touch
- Worse after sleep
- The remedy has a strong mental picture which needs consideration (talkative, often jealous and aggressive, also depressed and sad)

disturbed the snake shakes its tail, causing a loud rustling sound in the undergrowth. It is very aggressive, able to launch spontaneous attacks.

Habitat: The cool, moist undergrowth of the South American rain forests is the habitat of the Bushmaster.

Medicinal Action and its Uses: The poison of the snake acts as a coagulant on the blood and causes paralysis (restriction and cessation of movement) and haemorrhage. This shows as a purple discoloration of the skin where the bite was administered.

Therapeutics and Indications: The homoeopathic remedy Lachesis is gained by extracting the poison from the fangs of the snake. It is most useful in badly inflamed throats and female ailments. The former is indicated when the throat is very inflamed and swollen with a feeling of strangulation and constriction, worsened by the slightest touch. Curiously the throat symptoms are relieved by swallowing food but not liquid.

The back of the throat may appear with a purple or bluish discoloration. External pressure, such as a tight collar or necklace is unbearable. The left side of the throat is usually more affected or the symptoms start on the left and later move to the right.

In the female sphere, Lachesis is very beneficial in menstrual problems, severe abdominal pain before periods, PMT with mood swings etc. before the onset of menstruation, all *relieved immediately by the start of the flow*. Menopausal problems, like the common heat flushes and nocturnal sweating and palpitations can be treated successfully with Lachesis if the remedy is indicated. This may exceed home treatment and should be left to the professional practitioner.

Mentally the person likes to express him/herself verbally, Lach. patients are very talkative. They can be very jealous and aggressive, like the Bushmaster snake. They are sensitive to noise, touch and differences in temperature.

Potency and Dosage: In very sore throats with the feeling of constriction Lach. 30c, one dose, possibly with a second dose the following day should bring immediate relief. In female problems the same applies, Lach. 30c at the onset of the distressing symptoms will ensure a trouble-free cycle. However, if this is a recurrent problem, professional help from an experienced homoeopath should also be sought.

Ledum *(Plant)*
(Ledum palustre)

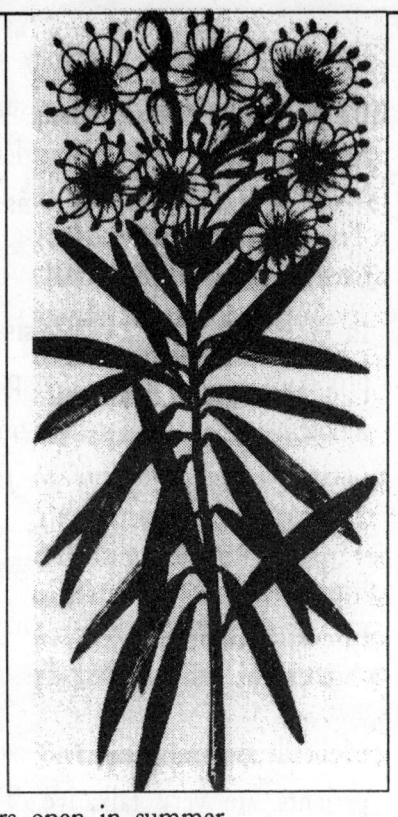

COMMON NAMES:
Marsh Tea,
Wild Rosemary

Description: A small evergreen shrub, 3-4 ft in height, native to Northern Europe, Canada and Greenland. The branches are woolly, as are the leaves on on the underside. White flowers open in summer.

Habitat: Ledum grows in cold bogs and mountain woods. When black tea was not available, Ledum was used as a substitute by the white settlers in North America. Ledum is a tough plant which has adapted well to its cold environment.

Medicinal Action and its Uses: The leaves have a spicy aroma and taste, which makes them useful as an insect and vermin repellent. Herbalists use extracts of the plant to treat coughs and inflamed membranes of the chest. Sore throats also seem to respond well to this treatment.

Therapeutics and Indications: Ledum is a valuable remedy in rheumatism, puncture wounds and insect bites. Puncture wounds caused by piercing with nails or needles, as well as bullet or shrapnel wounds and animal bites heal more quickly with a topical application of Ledum as a compress (5 drops/ ½ pint water). These type of wounds are cold to touch, yet curiously the cold also relieves the pain.

In rheumatic pains the joints are hot, swollen and painful. Heat is not tolerated, especially heat of the bed. The complaints start in the lower limbs and move upwards through the body. The beginning of any movement is particularly painful.

Potency and Dosage: Pierce wounds are best treated with diluted mother tincture (the undiluted extract of the plant). 5 drops of the tincture are added to a ½ pint of water and used as a compress. Rheumatic complaints, especially of a long-standing nature, respond best to Ledum 6c given for a week on a daily base.

Characteristics to remember:

- In puncture wounds and insect/animal bites Ledum prevents tetanus
- The wound is cold to touch
- Cold applications and a cool environment ameliorate these injuries
- Rheumatic pains start in the lower extremities and travel upwards
- Rheumatic pain is worse from the heat of the bed and at night

Mercurius Sol. *(Element)*

Mercurius Solubilis/ Vivus)

COMMON NAMES:
Mercury, Quicksilver

Description: Hg, Element 80, is silver in colour and unique among metals by being a liquid at room temperature, melting point is -39° Celsius, boiling point is 357° Celsius. The metal is used as temperature and pressure-measuring equipment. The vapour and soluble salts of the element are toxic.

Medicinal Action and its Uses: Formerly used to treat syphilis, it is now used as amalgam in dental fillings. Unfortunately dental patients can suffer from mercury poisoning when their fillings break down and the mercury leaks into the body. However, this is not always the case, depending on the stability of the compound and the sensitivity of the patient. Another danger lies in the mercury accumulated in the human body through the food chain and by inhaling the toxic fumes of mercury.

Therapeutics and Indications: Mercury destroys tissue as it is corrosive. The cells finally become unable to sustain life. As a homoeopathic preparation, Merc. sol. is an excellent remedy for skin problems and complaints associated with the digestive tract.

For home treatment one should concentrate on skin eruptions as in the case of acne, "spots" and possibly eczema, all of which are moist in nature and ooze yellow discharge. The eruption is also itchy and dislikes extreme heat or cold. The sufferer generally sweats a lot which brings no relief. The smell of the sweat is offensive. Generally the skin is oily/greasy rather than dry.

Inflamed and swollen tonsils with a sore throat is another good target for Merc. sol. if they burn and smart and exude yellow pus. The throat can be swollen and inflamed to such an extent that even swallowing liquid is an ordeal.

Fetid mouth odour is also common with this remedy.

All the above conditions are associated with night time aggravation and sensitivity to heat and cold.

Potency and Dosage: Merc. sol. 30c is the best potency for acute sore throats with the discussed associated symptoms: very swollen, exuding pus, worse at night and from hot and cold food and drinks. Long standing skin problems are best treated by the professional homoeopath but for home treatment Merc. sol. 6c, daily for a fortnight, should bring noticeable relief in skin problems which fit the remedy.

Characteristics to remember:

- In skin and tonsil problems
- always worse at night
- worse from extremes of temperature: heat and cold
- sweating is a critical area: too much, offensive smell, it aggravates the complaints
- ulcerating tonsils discharge yellow-green pus

Nat sulph. *(A Salt)*
(Natrum Sulphate)

Description: Chem. formula: $Na_2SO_4 \cdot 10H_2O$. This compound contains suphur and sodium, two very reactive elements, which were hydrated with H_2O (water).

> **COMMON NAMES:**
> *Glauber's salt,*
> *sulphate of sodium*

There are two ways of producing Glauber's salt: by strongly heating sodium chloride with concentrated sulphuric acid or by neutralising sodium hydroxide solution with sulphuric acid.

Glauber's salt was named after Johann Glauber (1604 - 1670), a follower of Paracelsus, who discovered sodium sulphate in 1668.

Medicinal Action and its Uses: Glauber's salt is one of Schuessler's original 12 tissue salts, it is a mild laxative (encouraging the voiding of the bowel) and it is present in many mineral waters. The effect of sodium sulphate is valued as an active compound in the bath- and drinking water of spas.

Therapeutics and Indications: Nat. sulph is a remedy indicated for home use in head injuries, especially for long-term effects of head injuries (after Arnica has been given).

Nat. sulph. is also useful in the treatment of asthma, although only with the help of a professional homoeopath, particularly if the asthma is chronic.

Head injuries which cause vertigo and headaches, loss of memory and epileptic convulsions can be treated with Nat. sulph. Arnica, a remedy also given for head injuries (p. 35) is an excellent first aid remedy to deal with the physical damage caused by the fall or blow (concussion), whereas Nat. sulph. deals with the physiological and psychological effects of such an injury.

Even if the trauma caused by the injury happened a long time ago, Nat. sulph. will clear up dizzy spells and "funny turns" relating to the accident.

The Nat. sulph. asthma always occurs in wet and damp weather, for example every spring or if there is a change from dry to wet weather. With the asthma attack there is often a soft bowel movement. The asthma is of the wet kind and produces thick discharges.

Potency and Dosage: In long-term effects of head injuries, depending on the severity of the symptoms, Nat. sulph. 6c or 30c given for five consecutive days, will bring noticeable relief.

Asthma which has been a long-term problem since childhood for example, should be treated with Nat. sulph. 6c, once a day for a fortnight. In recent asthma attacks which fit the description of Nat. sulph., a double dose of Nat. sulph. 30c (two tablets on two consecutive days) will clear up the symptoms considerably if not remove them completely.

Characteristics to remember:

- Asthma which is always worse from damp weather or change from dry to damp/wet
- Used to treat long-term effects of head injuries
- Music affects the emotional balance deeply and makes him/her sad
- Indicated in warm blooded, plump rather than skinny patients
- Any kind of damp: damp living conditions, damp weather, even food grown near water **aggravates**

Nux vomica (Plant)
(Nux Vomica)

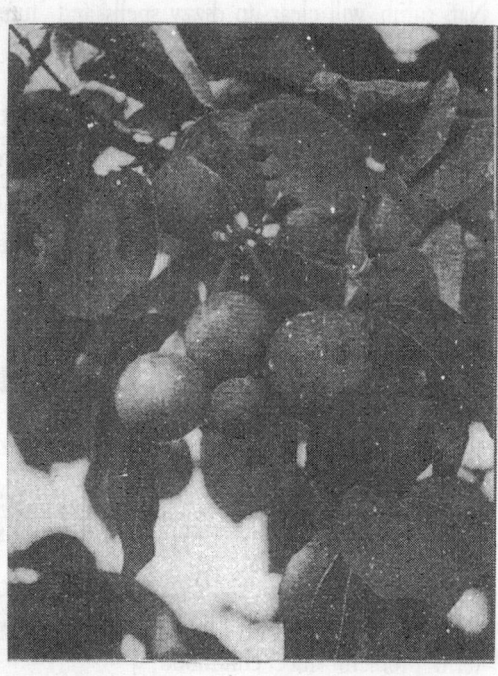

Description: Nux vom. is the seed from a medium sized tree with a short, thick trunk covered in ash-coloured bark, the Koochla tree. The wood obtained from this tree is hard and durable. The branches of the tree are irregular, the leaves are oval, nearly round, with each leaf opposite another. The flowers of the tree are small and green-white with an unpleasant smell. The fruit is about the size of a large apple with 5 seeds inside. The seeds are covered in fine satiny hair which give them a glossy sheen. They are very hard and have an extremely bitter taste.

COMMON NAMES:
Poison Nut

Habitat: The poison nut tree or Koochla tree (Strychnos nux vomica) is native to India and Sri Lanka, the East Indies, the Malay Archipelago and Northern Australia.

Medicinal Action and its Uses: Nux vom. contains alkaloids which act as a convulsive poison. After greatly exciting the reflex ability of the spinal cord, it finally kills the victim by paralysis of the central nervous system. In orthodox medicine these alkaloids have in small doses been used to treat bedwetting in children, as well as other debilities.

> **Characteristics to remember:**
>
> - Ill effects from over-indulgence in food, alcohol, other stimulants or recreational drugs
>
> - Cold and stimulants (coffee in particular) aggravate
>
> - Symptoms tend to be worse in the morning
>
> - Nux. vom. has particular mental and emotional characteristics

Therapeutics and Indications: The mother tincture (pure extract) of Nux vom. is prepared by using the seeds of the poison nut tree. In home prescribing Nux vom. is used successfully to treat hang-overs, stomach pain and headaches resulting from over-indulgence in food and/or alcoholic drink. As Nux vom. contains a very potent cocktail of poisons, Strychnine being one of them, it equally cures gastric disturbances, circulatory and sensory problems (headache, photophobia, dizziness and vertigo) resulting from such over-indulgence. It is therefore a good *morning after remedy*.

The patient feels worse from drinking coffee or taking any other stimulants. There is also aggravation after a meal. Cold, dry weather and cold conditions in general also aggravate. Morning is the worst time for the patient.

The remedy has very distinctive mental and emotional characteristics. The patient is likely to be easily irritated and impatient individual with the tendency to outbursts of violent temper. "Fools are not suffered gladly" could be the motto of the Nux vom. person, who is often highly competitive, a career person with little time to waste. On the other hand Nux vom. people are very sociable people who care about their friends and family. The tendency to over-indulge, however, is always present.

Potency and Dosage: In severe cases of hangover or symptoms related to such, one dose of Nux vom. 30c or 100c will alleviate promptly. If all the symptoms have not disappeared completely within the course of half a day, repeat the dose.

Extra tip: Ginger tea helps to overcome gastric upsets, see p. 60 (Ipecac) for instructions how to prepare the tea.

Paeonia (Plant)
(Paeonia)

> **COMMON NAME:**
> *Peony*

Description: A garden perennial with beautiful, often scented, opulent blooms. The plant grows to about 2 1/2 foot in height, the young leaves are reddish, later turning green and are divided into many segments. The fleshy roots are used for medicinal preparations, including homeopathy. Peony belongs to the family of Ranunculaceae, like the common buttercup and aconite, the latter used for another homeopathic preparation. Many cultivars of the plant are grown as ornamentals for the garden.

Habitat: Peony is a plant native to Europe, especially Greece. It is a long-lived plant when sited in the right conditions: deep, fertile soil, preferably manured every year. Full sun or slightly dappled shade is ideal.

Medicinal Action and its Uses: In herbalism, peony is used as an antispasmodic to treat nervous affections resulting in tics and convulsions. Formerly the powdered root was used to treat mania and hysteria.

Therapeutics and Indications: Paeonia has a special affinity to the rectum and the homeopathic preparation is used to treat haemorrhoids. If these are externally visible and very painful during and after stool they are best treated with Paeonia. There is much itching in the anus, which is swollen. Touch, like wiping after relieving oneself, aggravates the pain.

Potency and Dosage: Paeon. 6c or 30c, depending on the severity of the symptoms, taken three times a day for 2 to 3 days, will bring down the swelling and congestion. Paeonia as an ointment is also available for topical application.

Extra tip: A blend of essential oils, Frankincense, Juniper and Cypress, diluted to 2 drops of each into a 10ml bottle of carrier oil (grapeseed, olive, or almond oil) will help to reduce the swelling and pain. This preparation should be applied externally to the haemorrhoids at least 3 times daily.

There is also a homoeopathic preparation for external use (Cream) "Paeonia" available at the chemist.

Characteristics to remember:

- For external haemorrhoids
- Much itching and congestion of the anus
- Touch and pressure aggravates, such as cleaning oneself after stool
- Haemorrhoids may be fissured and covered with crusts

Pulsatilla (Plant)
(Anemone Pulsatilla) or (Pulsatilla vulgaris)

Description: Pulsatilla vulgaris is a perennial, growing in the wild in Britain and as a cultivated garden species. The plant is covered in fine downy hair, with a silvery appearance. It has woody, fibrous root stock and attains a height of 5-8 feet. The leaves are feathery, whereas the cup-shaped, nodding purple flowers with their yellow centre, approximately 1 1/2" in diameter, are the glory of the plant. Even the flowers, the under surfaces and outward facing sides of the petals, are covered in fine silky hair. The flowers appear in early spring.

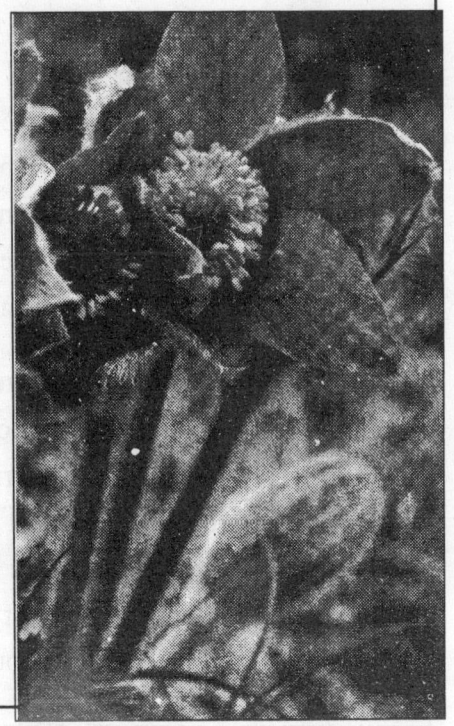

Habitat: Dry chalky soil, as in the chalk Downs of

> **COMMON NAMES:**
> *Pasque Flower,*
> *Wind Flower,*
> *Easter Flower*

the South East of England, is the preferred situation of this plant.

Medicinal Action and its Uses: Pulsatilla acts to reduce muscle spasm and therefore has been used to treat asthma, whooping cough and bronchitis. In herbalism it has also been used to treat problems relating to menstruation and the female cycle. The extract Anemonin, one of the active constituents of the chemical make-up of Pulsatilla, is a powerful irritant which can cause inflammation of the eyes and mouth. Equally, Anemonin causes gastro-enteritis when taken internally. It can be used to reduce the activity of the circulation, respiration and the nervous system.

Characteristics to remember:
- In PMT and menstrual problems
- In digestive complaints, mostly related to eating fatty food, esp. butter
- Eating aggravates the patient
- Drinks very little/not thirsty
- Patient is aggravated by heat and prefers the outdoors
- Distinctive mental/emotional picture

Therapeutics and Indications: Puls. is of great value in problems relating to the female cycle and digestive problems. PMT, delayed or scanty menstrual flow or very heavy flow can be treated with Puls. There is a sensation as if menstruation was imminent. Disorders of pregnancy, especially a tendency to miscarry and morning sickness, are commonly treated with Puls., but this should be left to the experienced homoeopathic practitioner.

Digestive problems which are related to fatty foods, such as food "repeating" after a meal, are common applications for this remedy. The abdomen is bloated, constipation is common and flatulence is a prominent feature. Eating in general aggravates the symptoms.

This remedy has distinctive mental/emotional characteristics. People who need Puls. are often female. They are very emotional and easily flip from one emotional state into another. They are easily moved and cry easily. They like support in the form of encouragement and sympathy, especially when ill. They will look for these qualities in others, their partner and friends, to fulfil their needs. However they also have a strong will of their own. Having made up their mind, they will pursue their goal, using "gentle" put persistent methods of persuasion.

Patients who need Puls. are said to be fair haired and blue eyed, but there are many exceptions to this rule!

Potency and Dosage: In PMT and menstrual problems, one Puls. 30c, morning and evening, prior to commencement of the period, will bring substantial relief. The same applies for digestive problems. Start with Puls. 30c and repeat once more if the symptoms have not disappeared within a day.

Rhus Toxicodendron *(Plant)*
(Rhus Toxicodendron)

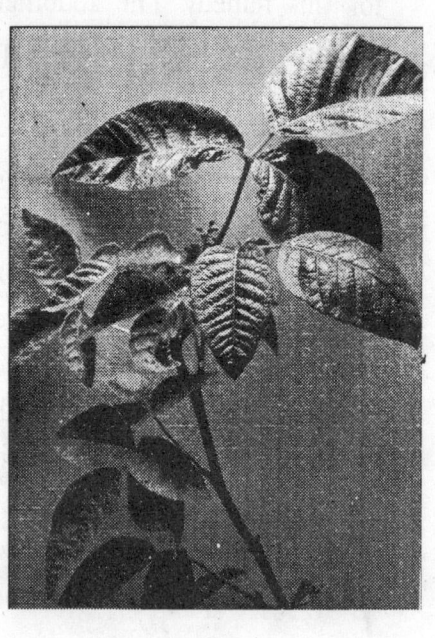

Description: Rhus tox. belongs to the genus of Rhus, which includes small trees, shrubs and shrubby climbers. Rhus tox. is a small shrub with ornamental foliage. The leaves are almost stalkless and indented, the flowers, which blossom in early summer, are green to yellow-white and small. The plant exudes an acrid sap, which is highly irritating.

Habitat: Rhus tox. grows in the thickets and undergrowth of North America, where it is common. The preferred position is sun and well-drained soil.

COMMON NAMES:
Poison Ivy,
Poison Vine,
Poison Oak

Medicinal Action and its Uses: The sap of the plant is a potent irritant which causes, when it comes in contact with the human skin, a severe rash with great swelling, intolerable pain and inflammation. The affected area subsequently ulcerates. Herbalists have used the plant for rheumatism and skin eruptions.

Therapeutics and Indications: Rhus tox. is an excellent homoeopathic preparation for the treatment of joint pain, incurred by sudden violent movement or by unusual strain. (Remember to give Arnica first). Backache also responds well to treatment with Rhus tox., especially, lower back pain. Stiffness and pain are relieved by movement, hence the name "rusty gate" remedy. Initially movement makes the sufferer feel better until the tearing or jerking pain and fatigue of the joint sets in again. Cold and wet

Characteristics to remember:

- For joint pains and backache, esp. of the lower back, from violent movement or unusual strain

- Pain and stiffness is significantly worsened by wet and cold, also by complete rest

- Symptoms are relieved initially from movement but pain returns after a short while

- Heat and hot applications, especially a hot bath, help

aggravates the symptoms severely. Rest, such as sitting, lying or even standing makes the pain and discomfort worse. Heat and hot wraps help to reduce the pain and stiffness. Rhus tox. rheumatism often comes on in the cold season of the year.

Potency and Dosage: Rheumatic complaints and joint pains in general are best treated with Rhus tox. 6c, twice daily for 3 days. Symptoms will have almost disappeared after this period, if there is some remaining pain and discomfort, continue treatment for another 4 days.

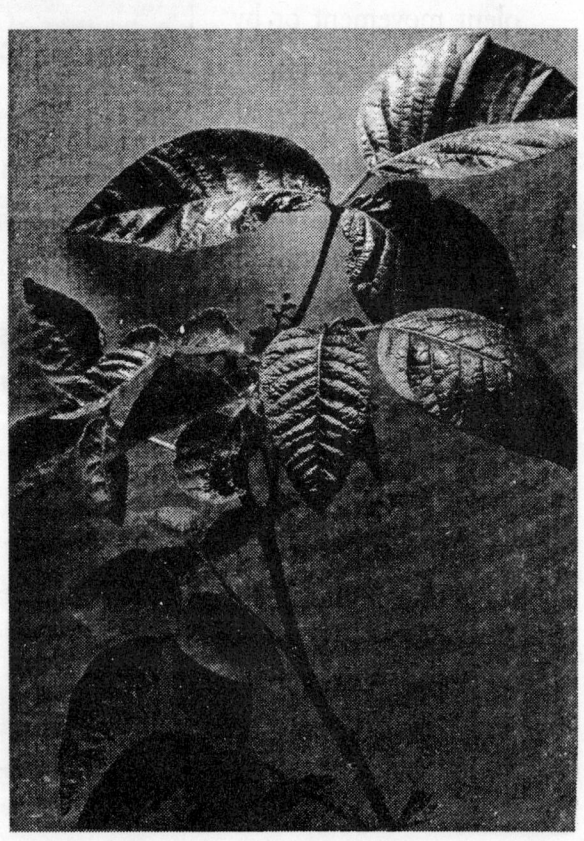

Ruta Graveolens (Plant)
(Ruta graveolens)

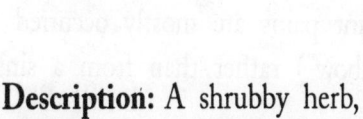

COMMON NAMES:
Rue, Garden rue, Herb-of-Grace

Description: A shrubby herb, attaining 20-80 cm in height. The leaves are feathery with a blue-green tint. The flowers, which appear between June and September are green-yellow. The whole plant emits a powerful, slightly unpleasant odour and possesses a very bitter, acrid taste.

Habitat: Rue prefers medium, dry soil. Chalk soil and a sunny situation offers perfect conditions.

Medicinal Action and its Uses: Rue has been used by ancient herbalists for its medicinal properties which promote digestion and stimulate the kidney. Rue's active ingredients, Rutin,

Characteristics to remember:

- For joint pains and backache from repetitive strain
- For tired eyes from over-straining
- Lame, bruised feeling all over, weariness
- Symptoms are worse from cold and wet, better from warmth

alkaloids, bitter agents and resins are beneficial for high blood pressure, headache, migraines etc. Rue also has a reputation for improving eye-strain and rheumatism.

Therapeutics and Indications: Ruta grav. is used homoeopathically for strains and sprains of the joints. It can be given as a second remedy after Arnica. The limbs and joints feel bruised, the tendons are sore and the joints may be swollen. Sciatic pain in the thighs and legs is better for walking up and down, worse for sitting or lying. Joint pains are mostly occurred by repetitive straining ("tennis elbow") rather than from a single injury.

Over-straining of the eyes, by reading small print, sewing or looking at a computer screen, is successfully treated by Ruta grav. The eyes are red and hot and are likely to be watery.

Care: The fresh plant is a powerful irritant and causes skin irritations.

Potency and Dosage: Joint pains and backache will be greatly relieved by Ruta grav. 6c, twice daily, morning and evening for three days. The symptoms will by then have improved drastically, but persistent pain and stiffness should be treated with Ruta grav. 6c, twice daily, for another 4 days.

Eye-strain should be treated with one dose of Ruta grav. 30c.

Symphytum (Plant)
(Symphytum Officinale)

Description: This herb has a short rootstock with black roots spreading outwards. They contain a very slippery, sticky substance.

> **COMMON NAMES:**
> *Common Comfrey, Boneset, Knitbone*

The leafy stem attains a height of 2-3 feet, is stout and hollow and covered with rough hair. The leaves are likewise covered in bristly hairs. They may cause itching when touched. The plant flowers from May to August, the flowers are set in opposite pairs along the stem, curving inwards ("scorpion's tail"). The bell-shaped flowers are dark violet/purple, with some forms displaying carmine red or yellow-white flowers.

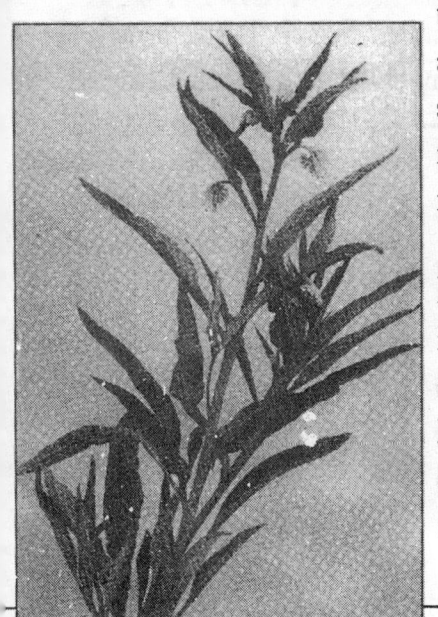

Habitat: Comfrey flourishes in damp places, especially along riverbanks, brooks and lakes. It also grows in meadows and beneath undergrowth along the margins of the forest. The plant is native to Europe and temperate Asia.

Medicinal Action and its Uses: Comfrey is renowned for its demulcent action, i.e. it promotes the production of viscid fluid which protects tender surfaces (lungs, bronchi, intestines, bones) from action of irritating substances or abrasive mechanical action. It is therefore given in cases of lung disease, whooping cough, inflammation of the respiratory tract and TB. Likewise it has been prescribed for intestinal ulcers and stomach ulcers and internal bleeding. Comfrey's "bone knitting" quality has been recognised when prescribing the herbal preparation for fractures and bruising. The name Symphytum derives its origin from the Greek word symphein (to bring together) and reflects the bone healing properties of the plant.

Therapeutics and Indications: In homoeopathy Symphytum is used for the treatment of fractures. Symph. is also beneficial for eye injuries caused by a blunt object. Use Symph. 6c in such cases daily for a week.

Potency and Dosage: In fractures, give Symph. 6c daily, one dose, for a week and then reduce the dose to every other day for a second week. In the third week limit the dose to two tablets of Symph. 6c.

Characteristics to remember:

- In fractures, promotes the healing of the bones
- For eye injuries, caused by a blow with a blunt object with bruising of the eyeball

Urtica Urens *(Plant)*
(Urtica Urens)

COMMON NAMES:
Stinging Nettle, Lesser Nettle

Description: The Lesser Nettle is a common roadside plant, it attains a height of 30 to 100 cm, well armed with stinging hairs all over the plant. The stinging action is the result of the fluid contained in the multitude of hairs. The Latin origin of Urtica urens, uro, which means to burn, allude to the stinging qualities of the plant and its homoeopathic use.

The leaves of the Lesser Nettle are oval, ending in a point, the white green flowers are small and unpretentious, are bunched together in long panicles resembling tiny necklaces.

Habitat: The Lesser Nettle is common to Britain and Northern and Central Europe. The plant is a frequent sight with few requirements as to the situation and soil.

Medicinal Action and its Uses: Young leaves of the Lesser Nettle are eaten in spring, to promote the "cleansing of the blood". One ingredient of the Lesser Nettle is iron, which makes the plant valuable as a food item. Generally, preparations of the Lesser Nettle are used for cleansing and detoxifying purposes, especially in spring and during fasting.

A common remedy is to cover painful joints with a poultice or plaster made from fresh nettle leaves. Infusions of the herb are said to increase hair growth.

Therapeutics and Indications: Urtica urens is of great value as a homoeopathic preparation for the treatment of insect bites and stings, minor burns and obviously nettle sting. The affected area stings and burns, there is numbness with red swelling. Urtica urens ointment is best for the quick treatment of these conditions. Topical applications can be applied according to the intensity and severity of the symptoms. A jar of Urtica urens cream on stand-by in the kitchen is very useful for minor burns and scalds.

Potency and Dosage: In the case of insect bites with severe burning and inflammation, Urtica urens 30c, one dose, will bring instant relief. Topical application of the cream is very beneficial in minor burns and scalds and in the rash caused by contact with stinging nettles.

Characteristics to remember:

- For insect bites and stings
- For minor burns and scalds
- In nettle rash caused by stinging nettles
- Symptoms are worsened by heat, touch and water

Veratrum album *(Plant)*
(Helleborus Album)

Description: The Christmas Rose, or White Hellebore, grows to nearly one and a half foot. Its names are derived from two Greek words hellin, to kill, and bora, food. The winter flowering time of this plant makes it very special, the yellow-white flowers with their yellow centres emerging just after Christmas, January to March. The blooms are beautiful 1-2 inches in diameter, with 5 petals to each bloom and a slightly nodding habit. The tough foliage is dark green with grey visible veins threading the leaf surface. The leaves have small spikelets along

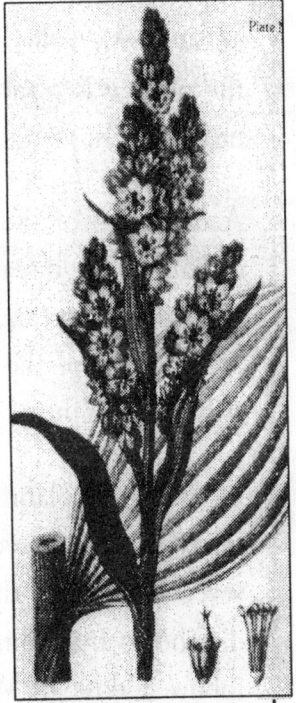

White hellebore, the source for Veratrum album. It was proved by Hahnemann and appears in the third volume of his Materia Medica Pura.

COMMON NAMES:
White Hellebore,
The Christmas Rose,
Weisse Nieswurzel

their edges. Altogether it is a beautiful plant and many garden cultivars are available.

Habitat: The White Hellebore prefers moist fertile, slightly limy soil. The plant resents root disturbance and is very long living once established. Helleborus Album is common in the mountains of Central and Southern Europe.

Medicinal Action and its Uses: All parts of the plant are highly poisonous. The Gauls were said to have rubbed their arrows with hellebore before the hunt. In medieval times the plant was regarded as a valid cure for insanity. Planted near the house the plant was said to ward off evil spirits.

A decoction of the plant was occasionally used to kill lice or cure skin diseases. It also found application for the treatment of mania, epilepsy etc. The ability to prolong the contractions of the heart has been put to good use in the treatment of heart disease.

However, the plant preparation is hardly ever used internally today due to its very poisonous nature. White Hellebore severely upsets the digestive system, causing profuse diarrhoea and vomiting. Violent pain and irritation will follow a dose of White Hellebore.

Therapeutics and Indications: The homoeopathic preparation, Verat., is completely safe to use in severe gastric upsets.

The marked characteristic is an icy coldness with cold sweat, especially on the forehead.

The digestive symptoms are: great thirst for cold drink, particularly water. The abdomen is contracted with excessive cramps which affect the whole body. The gastric upset causes vomiting and purging which leaves the patient completely weak and exhausted. The mouth feels dry, an intense nausea precedes the vomiting, the diarrhoea produced is copious, gushy, green and watery.

Verat. has been used in the treatment of cholera, yet this should better be left to the experienced practitioner.

The homeopathic preparation is also indicated in sudden violent temper tantrums and attacks of rage. Suddenly the individual becomes restless and destructive with the desire to break and

Characteristics to remember:

- Use in severe gastric upsets with vomiting, pain and purging
- Violent temper tantrums and attacks of rage are covered by this remedy
- The patient's face looks pale or bluish
- Pain compels the patient to move around
- Conditions are worse at night, from wet and cold weather
- Patient feels better when in cool environment

destroy objects. The patient is also very talkative, with a sometimes abusive, sometimes witty slant to his/her speech. This remedy can be indicated in violent moods during PMT, menstruation or pregnancy. This may also be the case in elderly patients, children or pets.

The careful home prescriber may identify these situations and recognize the remedy. However, an experienced homeopath should additionally be consulted, as these cases can be overwhelming and complex.

Potency and Dosage: In extreme attacks of gastric symptoms, one dose of Verat. 200c will make the violent bowel movement and vomiting cease. Follow-up with Verat. 30c if necessary. In emotional disturbances, violent moodswings, etc., one dose of Verat. 200c, should show some immediate positive results, yet professional advice is furthermore desired.

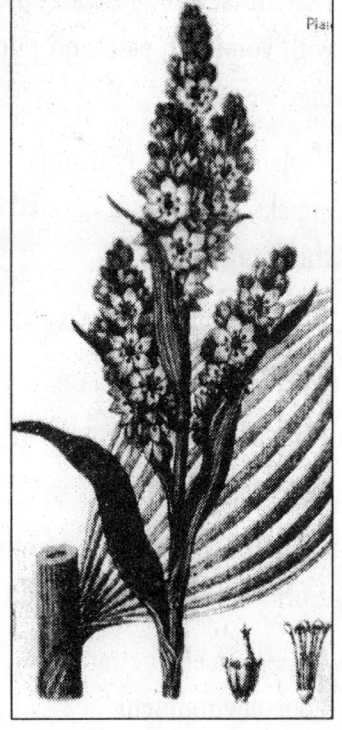

Index of Conditions and Symptoms

Accidents: Arn. p.37
Alcohol poisoning: Nux v. p.72
Asthma: Nat.sulph. p.70
Bronchitis: Bry. p.45
Backpain: Ruta grav. p.83, Rhus tox. p.80
Burns (minor): Urt.u. p.87
Catarrh: (Nose) All.c. p.33
Colds: Acon. p.31, Bell. p.41, Gels. p.57
Cystitis: Berb. p.43, Canth. p.49
Diarrhoea: Ars. p.39, Verat. p.89
Eye-strain: Ruta grav. p.83
Fever: Acon. p.31, Bell. p.41
Flatulence: Carb.v. p.51
Food poisoning: Ars. p.39, Verat. p.89
Fractures: Symph. p.85
Gallstones: Berb. p.43
Gastric upsets: Ars. p.39, Carb. v. p.51, Nux v. p.72, Verat. p.38
Hangover: Nux v. p.72
Hayfever: All.c. p.33
Haemorrhoids: Paeon. p.77
Headache: Gels. p.57, Nux v. p.72
Indigestion: Carb. v. p.51, Nux v. p.72

Influenza: Acon. p.31, Bell. p.41, Gels. p.57
Injuries: Any injury: Arn. p.37
      Head: Arn. p.37, Nat sulph. p.70
      Fingers/ Toes: Hyper. p.59, Spine: Arn. p.37, Hyper. p.59
Insect bites: Apis p.35, Urt.u. p.87
Joint pain: Arn. p.37, Ruta grav. p.83, Rhus tox. p.80
Menstrual cramps: Lach. p.63, Puls. p.77
Morning sickness: Ipec. p.61, Puls. p.77
Nausea: Cocc. (travel sickness) p.55, Ipec. p.61
Nettle rash: Urt.u. p.87
PMT: Lach. p.63, Puls. p.77
Rheumatism: Ruta grav. p.83, Rhus tox. p.80
Shock: Arn. p.37
Sore Throat: Lach. p.63, Merc. sol. p.68
Sunstroke: Bell. p.41
Temper tantrums: Cham. p.53, Verat. p.89
Teething problems: Cham. p.53
Tetanus prevention: Calen. p.47, Hyper. p.59
Tonsillitis: Lach. p.63, Merc. sol. p.68
Vomiting: Ars. p.39, Ipec. p.61, Verat. p.89
Wounds: Any type: Calen. p.47, Hyper. p.59
      Lacerated or puncture wound: Hyper. p.59, Led. p.66
      Large: Calen.p.47

Bibliography

Boericke, William *Pocket Manual of Homoeopathic Materia Medica*, Philadelphia, USA, 1927

Bricknell, Christopher(Ed.-in-chief) The Royal Horticultural *Society Gardeners' Encyclopedia of Plants and Flowers*, London 1989

Clarke, J.H. *Dictionary of Practical Materia Medica*, London, 1990

Crystal, David (Ed.) *The Cambridge Encyclopedia*, 2nd ed., Cambridge 1994

Cummings, Stephen & Ullman, Dana *Everybody's Guide to Homeopathic Medicines*, London, 1986

Gibson, Dr Douglas *Studies of Homoeopathic Remedies*, Beaconsfield, Bucks., 1987

Grieve, Mrs M F.R.H.S. *A Modern Herbal*, London 1931

Lexikon der Heilpflanzen, 2nd ed., Cologne, Germany, 1977·

Livingston, Ronald *Homoeopathy Evergreen Medicine*, Poole, 1991

Martin, Elizabeth A (Ed.) *Concise Medical Dictionary*, 3rd ed., Oxford, 1990

Vermeulen, Frans *Synoptic Materia Medica*, Haarlem, Netherlands, 1992.

DEDICATION

In dedication to all those who helped me on this journey, especially my friend Sarah and my husband John

Margit Wendelberger-James